It's Not All in Your Head

It's Not All in Your Head

Anxiety, Depression, Mood Swings, and Multiple Sclerosis

Patricia Farrell, PhD

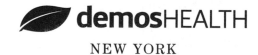

demosHEALTH

NEW YORK

Acquisitions Editor: Noreen Henson
Cover Design: Carlos Maldonado
Compositor: Absolute Service, Inc.
Printer: Hamilton Printing Company

Visit our Web site at www.demoshealth.com

Medical information provided by Demos Health, in the absence of a visit with a health care professional, must be considered as an educational service only. This book is not designed to replace a physician's independent judgment about the appropriateness or risks of a procedure or therapy for a given patient. Our purpose is to provide you with information that will help you make your own health care decisions.

The information and opinions provided here are believed to be accurate and sound, based on the best judgment available to the authors, editors, and publisher, but readers who fail to consult appropriate health authorities assume the risk of any injuries. The publisher is not responsible for errors or omissions. The editors and publisher welcome any reader to report to the publisher any discrepancies or inaccuracies noticed.

Library of Congress Cataloging-in-Publication Data

Farrell, Patricia.
  It's not all in your head : anxiety, depression, mood swings, and multiple sclerosis / Patricia Farrell.
       p. cm.
  Includes index.
  ISBN 978-1-932603-95-8
  1. Multiple sclerosis—Psychological aspects. 2. Multiple sclerosis—Patients—Mental health. 3. Multiple sclerosis—Complications. 4. Depression, Mental. 5. Anxiety. I. Title.
  RC377.F37 2011
  616.8'34--dc22

                              2010038314

Special discounts on bulk quantities of Demos Health books are available to corporations, professional associations, pharmaceutical companies, health care organizations, and other qualifying groups. For details, please contact:

Special Sales Department
Demos Medical Publishing
11 W. 42nd Street
New York, NY 10036
Phone: 800–532–8663 or 212–683–0072
Fax: 212–941–7842
E-mail: rsantana@demosmedpub.com

Made in the United States of America

11 12 13   5 4 3 2

Contents

Preface

This book is intended for anyone with a diagnosis of multiple sclerosis (MS) who has to live with the anxiety and depression from it as well.

When researching this book, one statement I came across really summed up the relevance of testing and of getting a definitive diagnosis on depression. It was the researcher's opinion that only one question was needed and that was, "Are you depressed?" It was simple and to the point and 94% of the people who responded "Yes" were, in fact, found to be depressed upon further evaluation.

I have had many years of direct clinical and research experience and have been fortunate to have been trained by some exceptional professionals. This training has led me to understand that we are each truly the best judges of our own illnesses. So you are the best person to answer the question "Are you depressed?"

As one physician with whom I worked said to a patient, "You know your body best." It may not always seem that way to others, but our experience of our lives is unique and, therefore, cannot be categorized into a set of numbers and test results.

In this book, you'll see several people I interviewed who knew their bodies, but had to try very hard to convince professionals that there was "something wrong" before they got their diagnosis of MS. It is a tribute to their courage and motivation to work toward health and, I hope, an inspiration for readers. As you'll see, sometimes you just have to trust your instincts.

I believe that if you wish to take several tests to get an "official" diagnosis of depression and/or anxiety, this can be accomplished quite easily on the Internet. Some of the self-test sites out there are supported by well-known, major medical and research institutions, and I urge you to seek them out if you truly wish to take some tests. Most of the tests taken prior to having an in-person clinical evaluation by a mental health professional and offered by reputable sites will indicate if you suffer from depression.

It is my intention with this book to help people living with MS to self-direct themselves to help alleviate some of the emotional symptoms related to MS. Although not a substitute for one-on-one therapy, I believe this book can be an important addition to both understanding MS and utilizing some of the tools that research has shown to be especially helpful in autoimmune disorders relative to anxiety, depression, and quality of life. One area of special note and where research is especially exciting is exercise, and I've provided a sterling example of one person who has fought the odds of his primary progressive MS with amazing results. Again, he's one individual, but new studies correlating exercise with the lessening of symptoms of MS are popping up every day.

The book starts with a basic understanding of MS as an autoimmune disorder and what that entails. It then continues with the workings of the central nervous system and how that relates to MS and the usual accompaniment of anxiety and depression for persons with MS. Also included are chapters on the things that you can do to help yourself, on looking forward to the future in terms of research and research breakthroughs, as well as a section that provides names and Web sites for organizations, books, and articles that will provide further information and assistance for people living with MS.

Actual people with MS have been interviewed for this book, and have discussed their methods of coping with living with MS. We've also included interviews with researchers in the area of MS and depression, and several techniques that research has shown to be helpful regarding depression, anxiety, and the immune system.

The book is not intended to be technical and difficult to understand, nor do I engage in anything near psychobabble. I am a proponent of using easily understood ways to tackle complicated ideas.

We know that MS is not "all in your head," as one patient said to her treating physician. It is a chronic illness that brings with it biologically driven psychological changes. These changes can often be difficult to endure but they are not totally psychological. There are, of course, psychological changes associated with accepting the diagnosis and resulting changes in functioning relative to any chronic illness, but you are not helpless here, either. We know that this is a "two-way disorder" and that anything you can do in terms of your thinking about the disorder and self-help will benefit you.

The basic aim of the book, therefore, is to provide concrete ways to help you help yourself psychologically and, in turn, your immune system. The connection between the two is, I believe, now fairly well-established. Therefore, anything you do for yourself in terms of lessening anxiety, depression, and stress is going to benefit you psychologically and physically.

As one woman thoughtfully said to me, "I have MS but MS does not define me." It does not define you, either.

Acknowledgments

Books are never the product of one person or of one writer's efforts, but rather they are the efforts of all those who participated in interviews and provided access to their innermost thoughts and concerns, who provided direction for the writer in terms of research, life stories, or just things that needed to be considered. A book, therefore, is a collaborative effort and to fail to acknowledge this would be unacceptable for me or for any writer.

Special thanks go to the physicians, researchers, psychologists, organizational staff, and writers, including (in alphabetical order) Debby Bennett, George Bonanno, Nancy Chazen, Nancy Chiaravalloti, Jeffrey Cohen, Jeffrey Gingold, Stefan Gold, Rosalind Kalb, Lauren Krupp, Rita D. Posner, Ruchika Prakash, Robert Sapolsky, Randolph Schiffer, and countless others worldwide who graciously shared their thoughts, articles, and research papers with me without question. I am truly amazed that they did so, unhesitatingly, when they heard my book's topic. In fact, their e-mail responses were returned within hours and sometimes within minutes of my requests, with papers attached. Yes, I was and am truly amazed by their generosity and the speed of their responses. I am also thankful to the staff of The National Multiple Sclerosis Society for their help with my research and the interviewing process.

Also, I am grateful for the encouragement and assistance of Noreen Henson, who pursued a book idea after I made a presentation at an MS consortium meeting. I believe she knew my heart was in the project and she continued her contact with me until I found myself available. It has been a labor of love and one of incredible learning for me.

It's Not All in Your Head

1

Multiple Sclerosis Made Simple

Multiple sclerosis (MS) is a neurodegenerative disorder of the central nervous system (CNS), meaning it affects the brain, spinal cord, and optic nerves, all of which comprise the CNS. The process is thought to be caused by an attack of the body's immune system on the delicate covering on nerves and areas of the brain related to mood, memory, judgment, concentration, and movement.

You will often hear people living wih MS talk about concentration problems as well as memory difficulties, which they have referred to as "brain fog." In one survey, more than 9,000 people with MS reported brain fog. The most common symptom reported in this non-scientific survey was fatigue, reported by more than 10,000 people living with MS. Even more illuminating, survey participants together reported an astounding 2,433 symptoms associated with their MS, which points to how such a wide symptom array can lead to confusion in the diagnosis. Those with less common symptoms may find themselves going to a succession of health care providers before they ultimately get the correct diagnosis.

MS has been termed a "communication breakdown" between the various parts of the nervous system triad and the body as a whole. Normal CNS functioning requires that electrical signals be sent to the spinal cord and the optic nerves from the brain and return signals are sent from the body to the brain through the spinal cord and the optic nerves in a two-way communication process.

When there is a communication breakdown, there is a host of associated physical and mental symptoms. Both types of disruptions result from MS, and these symptoms, unfortunately, can fluctuate so often that it may be difficult to diagnose the disorder. Some individuals have such subtle problems that they dismiss them and may go for years before a diagnosis is made.

MS can progress to the point that the person living with the disease can no longer work. But some people with an MS diagnosis may have no more than a few flare-ups their whole lives. Other people with MS may experience a progressive or relapsing form of the disorder.

The Symptoms

Symptoms of MS are varied and, for that reason, may not immediately be noticed as being related to the disorder. Some of the most obvious and common symptoms associated with MS include the following:

1. Muscle weakness
2. Spasticity
3. Impairment in sensitivity to temperature, touch, or pain
4. Pain (moderate to severe)
5. Ataxia or unsteady gait
6. Tremor
7. Speech disturbances
8. Vision disturbances
9. Vertigo
10. Bowel and bladder dysfunction
11. Sexual dysfunction
12. Depression
13. Euphoria
14. Cognitive changes such as concentration or memory problems
15. Fatigue

As noted by the National Institute of Neurological Disorders and Stroke (NINDS), the symptoms of MS are varied and not all of them may be present in one individual. It is this variance as well as the waxing and waning of symptoms that have often caused delayed diagnosis and treatment of MS in the past. Researchers, however, have developed new and more sophisticated methods that now provide more accurate means of assessment; treatment can begin sooner, thus possibly preventing further injury to the CNS.

Cognitive Impairment

In all of the symptoms noted, impairment in cognition appears to be the one that most people worry the least about until it happens to them. What constitutes this *cognition* problem?

Cognition is primarily composed of the higher functioning activities of the brain, which are involved in:

1. The ability to learn
2. Memory
3. Organizational skills and planning
4. Maintenance and shifting of attention, as needed
5. The use of appropriate language
6. Perceiving what's happening in our environment
7. Ability to do simple calculations and engage in financial activity

MS affects all of these abilities as well as reading comprehension. All of our information processing skills (the senses of vision, hearing, touch, smell, and taste), when impaired, can have a significant effect on our ability to function as we once did. For some people, the impairment may be minimal; for others, it can be much more debilitating and can affect walking and memory in a major way.

Consider how you would be affected by the impairment of your ability to recall words and to engage in normal social or career interactions. Picture yourself in a group, actively listening to a conversation, and then someone turns to you for a comment and you find you are unable to provide something reasonable. What would happen if you suddenly lost your train of thought, forgot what you wanted to say, and then couldn't express yourself? One man described it as "word fishing" and, for him, it is a serious problem. Would you begin to withdraw from social interactions, and would others begin to wonder what was happening to you?

For other people living with MS, it's not just word-finding problems that bring on additional difficulties; balance is a significant problem in their MS. There was a famous entertainer who had this problem. No one knew about the MS and, until this person received the diagnosis, there were major problems walking and maintaining balance. Workers on film sets and in hotels began to pass the word around that this person was an alcoholic. Not wanting to let the diagnosis out, even when it had been definitively made, the entertainer kept it secret from everyone, including close friends. Believe it or not, the stigma of being seen as an alcoholic seemed a preferable alternative to the diagnosis of MS.

The thought was that, if people who did the hiring in the industry learned of the MS, there would be no jobs or fewer jobs for this person. Insurance companies would refuse to provide coverage for films and, if there were no coverage and no guarantee to the film's backers, the film wouldn't be made. It took several years of less and less work until the decision was finally made to reveal the condition to the general public. At that point, major physical changes had taken place and this person had no reason to want to continue with a career. Fortunately, membership in a major entertainment trade union with good health care coverage and a pension made up for the loss of the career income.

Undoubtedly, stigma plays a major part in the lives of everyone with MS because there is still not enough knowledge about this disorder. There is no reason for anyone with MS to be ashamed because, as you will hear from health care professionals and those living with the condition, they did nothing wrong. It's just something that happened.

Today, thanks in large part to the advances in treatments, the physical disabilities that go along with the disease are becoming less and less severe. Within the larger group, the main functions of general intellect, remote or long-term memory, simple conversational skills, and reading comprehension also appear to suffer from less impairment.

There may be difficulty in making decisions or an impulsivity that begins to appear. Routines may no longer seem so simple to adhere to as they once were. Instructions are heard but not adequately processed, and carrying them out increases in difficulty. This, in turn, feeds back and there begins work dysfunction, problems in relationships, and personal esteem. But these come on gradually, not overnight.

How these changes come about is not the same for everyone. Some current research, in fact, is pointing to more than one type of MS that may account for the changes and the differences in benefit from standard treatments. There are individuals who will see subtle changes in some of these abilities and may dismiss it as being tired or the effect of too little sleep or poor diet. They may, however, have had a problem with low-level depression prior to their diagnosis of MS and this may have caused them to believe that their cognitive changes were caused by the depression or possibly some medication they were taking.

But what causes the symptoms and this lack of neural communication, you may be asking, and how common is it? Who gets the disorder and what kinds of things can be done to diagnose or treat it? First, let's look at some statistics on the illness in order to place it in some perspective regarding who gets MS and how many people have it.

What Is Multiple Sclerosis?

According to NINDS, MS was first diagnosed in 1894, but probably existed prior to that date. The disease generally shows up between the ages of 20 and 40 years and is more common in women, who are diagnosed at twice the rate of men. MS can also be found in children, so it is not strictly a disorder confined to adults.

Although there have been various theories put forth, the probable cause of MS is still being actively researched. The most prominent theory, at this time, is that it is one of the autoimmune disorders in which cells in the body that are supposed to protect us act in an abnormal fashion. In other words, instead of protecting the individual from "invaders" such as bacteria, infection, viruses, fungi, and parasites, the cells begin to attack a portion of the nervous system. The cells fail to recognize the person's cells as "friendly" and instead see them as "enemy" cells. Our internal defenders run amok and fail to perform their predetermined function.

Most of the damage is to a specific portion of the nervous system, which is at the heart of nerve communication. The parts of our CNS that are attacked include both the delicate, fatty covering over the nerve pathways that are necessary for normal nervous system functioning and the brain itself.

The covering on the nerves protects the communication highway for all movement and thought. If nerve cells cannot communicate with or "talk" to each other, the result is a disability in some function performed by those specific cells under attack.

Let's take a look at one portion of the nervous system that is involved and the structures that are included in the areas this disorder attacks. Admittedly, this is a highly simplified explanation of this intricate, still inadequately understood, disorder.

The Three Major Components

As mentioned previously, the three major components that make up the CNS are the brain, the spinal cord, and the optic nerves, which are actually stalks of the brain. All communication within this system is made possible by electrical and chemical changes initiated by changes in levels of two electrolytes (potassium and sodium) within the nervous system. Chances are you've had your electrolytes checked regularly during your annual physical exam as part of the blood work, because electrolytes are important barometers of your body's health.

If you've ever gone on a weight-reduction diet in which you lost too much potassium, then you have experienced several of the symptoms of nerve conduction disruption such as anxiety, depression, insomnia, and even suicidal thinking. This is a clear example of what happens when this potassium–sodium balance is upset.

These two electrolytes, in fact, play a vital role in all nerve conduction. Slight changes in the level of potassium and sodium can contribute to major changes in mood, anxiety, and even perception.

Let's leave the realm of biology for a moment and think of the entire system in a way that's much more familiar to you. Think of it in terms of a computer or any electrical gadget in your home and the electrical power cord for the computer or gadget that is inserted into the electrical outlet in the wall. Imagine the computer as your brain. In many ways, your brain is an extremely sophisticated computer and, as well, a chemical factory that manufactures powerful chemicals called *neurotransmitters*.

The electrical cord that plugs into the wall, which supplies electricity to the computer, has an insulating covering on it to both protect you from the electricity in the wires and to help the electricity in the cord go from the wall to the computer. In our CNS, the electricity actually goes two ways: from the brain (i.e., the computer in my example) to the electrical power cord and from portions of our nervous system back to the brain. Both the power cord and your nervous system's axons (the major pathways in the nervous system) in your body work in a very similar fashion with one exception. The exception is that your axons (see Figure 1.1) produce their own "electricity" by way of chemical reactions. Remember the potassium and sodium I mentioned before? Well, what's causing the electrical changes here?

The Healthy Neuron

Figure 1.1 shows a simplified nerve cell, much like the ones that would be attacked by MS.

Each neuron is made up of, basically, five fundamental parts:

1. **Cell body**, responsible for maintaining the health and functioning of the cell
2. **Axon** or "cable"
3. **Node of Ranvier**, the tiny space between cells *on the axon*
4. **Myelin sheath** (the fatty material made up of Schwann cells), which coats and protects the axon
5. **Dendrites**, which reach out like roots from the axon to muscles, glands, or other neurons and allow communication to other nerve cells

The protective material on the neuron's axon is called the **myelin sheath**. Myelin is a fatty material that is wrapped around the axon just

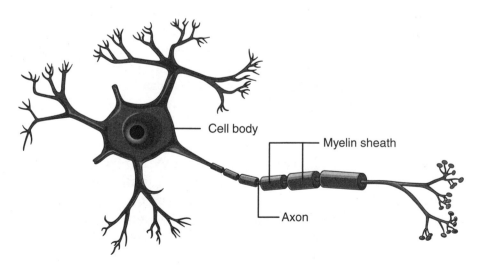

Cell body

Myelin sheath

Axon

Figure 1.1 A healthy neuron.

as the insulating material is wrapped around the electrical power cord of your computer. The one interesting difference is that the myelin on your neuron's axons is made up of a series of little links that look like "sausage links." The incredibly tiny space between each link, called the **node of Ranvier**, actually helps speed the transmission of the electrical charge in your nervous system as it jumps the gap. This jumping action helps move the charge even faster.

These little spaces help those electrical pulses move incredibly fast and facilitate the movement of your limbs, your thought processes, speaking, walking, and several other things. They also allow you to perform physical actions and mental activity smoothly and, sometimes, very rapidly. When there is a lack of smoothly executed muscle movement, this can indicate a problem in this "link" system between the brain, the eye, or the spinal cord. One example of problematic smooth movements is seen in the eye movements of patients with MS. It is often a diagnostic indicator of MS or a nerve problem known as *internuclear ophthalmoplegia* (INO) in which the eyes do not track smoothly and may have a jerky movement when looking toward the extreme right or left.

On the axon, each sausage link or Schwann cell, in fact, wraps itself around the axon, much like the layers of an onion. This protective layer allows a series of inflow and outflow actions by the electrolytes in your axons. Electrical impulses caused by this flowing-in-and-out action allow an electrical charge to come down from the brain through the axon and out to muscles and glands. It is one of the marvels of the human body, and a similar action takes place on the way back from the muscles and glands. The problems in MS are caused by destruction of that insulating material, the myelin sheath, which causes a rupture in the electrochemical transmission of information from the brain to parts of the body. These injuries to the myelin sheath are thought to be caused by some malfunctioning of the immune system, which initiates an inappropriate attack on the sheath by specialized cells.

These specialized blood cells begin to destroy a portion of the myelin sheath, which then results in problems in the electrical conduction I mentioned earlier. The extent of the destruction varies and that is what causes anything from mild, moderate, and up to severe damage to the sheath. The result is impairment in movement or glandular action. In the brain, a similar form of destruction would cause scarring, which can affect memory, concentration, mood, or judgment, depending on where the injury takes place.

The Damaged Neuron

Figure 1.2 illustrates how an area of the axon's myelin sheath, when destroyed, stops that electrical charge from reaching its destination at the end of the axon. It's at that endpoint where the charge would have passed chemicals (neurotransmitters) on to another neuron, gland, or muscle. The *demyelinated area* is clearly shown in Figure 1.2.

Dr. Randolph Schiffer, director of the Cleveland Clinic Lou Ruvo Center for Brain Health, Las Vegas, Nevada, has said:

> Our understanding of MS is changing because of new research in the field. We know that patients with MS in its early stages can have a variety of responses to the disease. Some have a relapsing and remitting course and for some people it stays that way. But for others it can change over time to a progressive sort of disease in which not only white matter (the axons) but also gray (brain cells) matter structures are affected and harmed.

This damage is often referred to as *plaque formations* or *scarring*.

"The word plaque in MS is from an old French word that meant a hard thing like a shell and it's a scar caused by specialized cells. This scarring prevents the nerve cells from communicating with each other and this can contribute to the cognitive impairment," explains

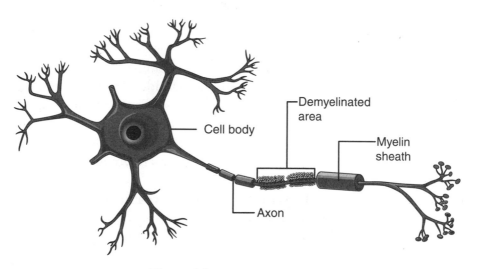

Figure 1.2 A damaged neuron.

Dr. Schiffer. There are brain cells, called *glial cells*, or *oligodendro-cytes*, that actually lay down new myelin and others that cause scar-ring. This repair function of those specialized cells may indicate the promise of new and innovative treatments, and that is one hopeful area of current investigation. Stem cells research, as you will see later in the book, is also being investigated as a potential source of repair.

Dr. Schiffer maintains an optimistic outlook for anyone with MS: "The news is really good if you have the disease now because, while we don't have cures, in fact cures in medicine are extremely rare for cer-tain serious diseases, but for the most part we improve our treatments one step at a time. In MS we've done very well." And the improvements continue to come in terms of new treatments. Dr. Schiffer is currently involved in a treatment protocol that involves antidepressant me-dication and psychotherapy, which he hopes will further improve treat-ment options.

"There's very sophisticated science now with new treatments being approved every three to five years. Yes, that's a long time if you have the disease, but in terms of other diseases, like Alzheimer's, where we've gone 20 years with not much improvement in treatments, we're doing very well." In terms of what can be done by the patient, Dr. Schiffer said, "It could be that being positive and actively working to combat depression may be favorable for the long-term course of the disease."

Anger and Multiple Sclerosis

Research has shown that MS has physical and cognitive effects, and two of the latter are related to memory and anger. A 2009 research study, which included people with both relapsing–remitting and pro-gressive MS, pointed to how anger alone, outside of any influence of anxiety or depression, might be "a direct consequence of the demyeli-nation of the connections" between brain centers controlling anger and judgment. Although this may be a process of MS, it does not mean that you should give up and give in to it, but it points to yet another aspect of the disorder that needs to be managed.

One of the other findings of this study was that much of the anger felt by patients with MS was withheld, which, researchers suggested, can be associated with a negative impact on a person's physical health, espe-cially in terms of blood pressure and vascular disorders. Unfortunately, researchers noted that many times, this anger is not adequately explored by clinicians with the patient and, because it is withheld, is not noted because it doesn't show up in all their social/familial interactions.

We've often heard that "anger not dealt with" can cause a series of medical problems and when you have a serious disorder to begin with, it can only do more harm. Therefore, in the coming chapters, you will see how you can begin to change how you express your thoughts and how to develop new coping skills, both verbal and physical. Yes, physical, as you will soon see.

Depression, Anxiety, and Mood Swings

A symptom that is another common aspect of MS is its effect on mood dysfunction, which brings on depression or elation resulting in unexpected or inappropriate mood swings. Mood swings are characterized by unexpected and sudden shifts in mood that are uncharacteristic of the person's usual mood. These may include outbursts of anger, almost out of the blue and out of all proportion to what's happening, aggressive behavior regarding inconsequential matters, and there may even be a sense of euphoria in which unrealistic plans are made or major changes in lifestyle are seen as viable.

Multiple studies of patients with MS have indicated a high prevalence rate for depression in patients, with some estimating that 50% or more may have mood disturbances. Experts in the area of MS and depression believe the number may even be higher and note that it is a common characteristic of most, if not all, autoimmune disorders.

Typically, researchers found a high degree of anxiety among those with both MS and mood disorders. Some of these studies have mixed results but do indicate that there may be an important social aspect to depression in patients with MS that has been overlooked. Social factors can play a vital role in the development of depression, and both coping styles and social support are seen as being instrumental in helping patients with MS deal with the ensuing depression and anxiety they experience.

What are the major symptoms of anxiety anyone would experience whether they had MS or not? It may sound like a simple question, but it is surprising how the symptoms can be quite broad and can be missed as anxiety per se. Anxiety disorders are fraught with both physical and psychological reactions. Among the physical symptoms are those typically found when running for your life, which include sweating, nausea, problems in breathing, heart palpitations, trembling, either hot flashes or cold chills, muscle pain or tension, numbness, dizziness, fatigue, a feeling of restlessness, and gastrointestinal problems such as constipation or diarrhea. Some people even experience a great deal of discomfort trying to swallow food when there is no evidence that they have any physical problem that would cause such a problem.

The psychological symptoms of anxiety are more easily recognized and include feelings of apprehension or fear, constant worry, foreboding that something bad is about to happen, a fear of losing control, irritability, uneasiness, difficulty concentrating, negative thoughts, a fear of dying, feeling detached from things almost as though they were unreal, and panic. Not all of these will be felt by any one person and they represent various anxiety disorders, and it should be kept in mind that many people do have more than one anxiety disorder.

When we talk about a feeling of foreboding or of losing control, it is usually without a basis in reality. There may be no reason to be apprehensive or for you to fear that you'll lose control, but that's how anxiety makes you feel; it removes your sense of confidence that you can handle things. And it becomes a self-perpetuating problem as it makes you feel uneasy in situations in which you've experienced any of these problems before. So, anxiety ties a knot around you mentally and physically, and MS can be right there helping to pull it tighter unless steps are taken to constrain it.

Think about how either anxiety or depression can affect your ability to function and to do the things you need to do or enjoy doing. I remember a young student who, in the throes of an anxiety attack, lost her place in a multiple-choice exam sheet. The test was intended for entry into gifted and talented programs, so the stress of doing well plus a preexisting tendency toward anxiety and low-level depression both worked against the student. This is what can happen to students who have MS; they have problems remaining on task, concentration becomes problematic, and the added stress only exacerbates the problem. If left untreated or undiagnosed, it can have a major impact on their schooling and their career choices. We'll see more about adolescent or pediatric MS later in this book where we've interviewed one of the experts in the field.

Initial Screening for Depression

The student mentioned earlier could have benefitted from psychotherapy, which has been shown to be effective for depression alleviation when it is focused on coping skills rather than insight-oriented therapy. The question that remains for many researchers: Why isn't every person with MS routinely screened for depression and anxiety? Initial evaluation could lead to speedy treatment to lift this mood disorder. Considering the serious consequences on other aspects of the patient's functioning (e.g., concentration, memory, social involvement, maintenance of therapeutic treatments), it would seem that people with MS need an assessment for depression, anxiety, and anger management.

The question of lack of screening and treatment becomes even more urgent when it is considered that younger persons diagnosed with MS may be at higher risk of suicide because of their resulting depression. The standard protocol these researchers emphasize, therefore, includes a depression screening test in all evaluations for MS.

There is an additional feeling of helplessness that comes as a symptom of depression and, when joined with the diagnosis of MS, may be an important contributing factor to changes in quality of life. Targeted therapies that provide the patient with more adequate means to deal with their illness have been suggested as providing more beneficial results. A number of these issues will be dealt with in the following chapters of this book where we include self-help techniques that are varied and suited for many situations.

Memory Impairment

Memory or cognitive impairment appears to be a common symptom in MS and presents additional challenges to those with MS and those who are providing treatment to them. This impairment in working (short-term) memory, according to some studies, appears to be related to depression and, possibly, fatigue. Anything that will alleviate depression may have a positive effect on memory enhancement. If you consider that depression affects motivation, concentration, social interactions, and even fatigue, it is fairly easy to see how decreasing depression could provide a boost to memory and lifestyle.

Methods for memory enhancement are actively pursued in rehabil-itation and research facilities and many of these can be used at home as self-help aids. These are dealt with in the succeeding chapters in this book where we include many tips on how you can learn to cir-cumvent some of the memory problems you've been experiencing. I especially like a technique called *self-generated memory* and I think most people will find that one very helpful. The researcher who intro-duced it to me told me that she uses this technique herself and she doesn't have MS.

The Social Side of Multiple Sclerosis

The social side of MS is an area that does require attention both from anyone with MS and anyone who is treating or involved in the life of a person living with MS. We are social creatures and although some of us may be more social than others, it still remains necessary to learn to contain our emotions, get our wishes across to others, and engage in normal, pleasant interactions. Of course, if there is some degree of disability in your MS, you'll want to work closely with someone like your spouse, partner, or caregiver. Their social support is not only vital to you, but it's also a health-promoting interaction because social support can decrease stress, and stress, by most accounts, needs to be managed and contained.

One study indicated that levels of pain in women with MS were related to quality of life in which social support can play an impor-tant role in decreasing pain. Pain, as studies have shown, seems to share the same nerve pathways as fatigue and pain is also related to levels of anxiety. If you can decrease anxiety, or increase enjoy-able social interactions, then you can affect not only levels of pain but fatigue and depression as well. Picking up a few tips on improv-ing social interactions has a far-reaching effect in terms of other aspects of MS.

A diagnosis of MS implies the beginning of a journey. The journey may have already begun for you, and it's our hope that we can make it a bit smoother and more comfortable for you.

We only ask that, if you have MS, you keep an open mind about what you can do for yourself now, not what things you can no longer do as well as you once did. Optimism and being open to trying new things, even if you are a bit reluctant, make you part of the solution to getting help. You can make things happen, so we ask that you remember that. I am something of a coach in some of the chapters and that's because I think everyone needs reassurance and help in keeping up one's motivation. Every day won't be a good one, but you can make it a better day for you.

Further Reading

Cummings JL, Ariniegas DB, Brooks BR, et al. Defining and diagnosing involuntary emotional expression disorder. *CNS Spectrs*. June 2006;11(6):1–7.

Feinstein A. An examination of suicidal intent in patients with multiple sclerosis. *Neurology*. 2002;59(5):674–678.

Gingold JN. *Facing the Cognitive Challenges of Multiple Sclerosis*. New York: Demos Medical Publishing; 2006.

Goldberg S. *Clinical Neuroanatomy Made Ridiculously Simple*. 3rd ed. Miami: MedMaster, Inc; 2003.

Holland NJ. *Clinical Bulletin Information for Health Professionals: Overview of Multiple Sclerosis*. New York: National Multiple Sclerosis Society; 2006.

Macher J, ed. Neuropsychiatric manifestations in neurodegenerative disease. *Dialogues Clin Neurosci*. 2007;9(2). Available at: http://www.dialogues-cns.org. Accessed December 20, 2009.

McKinley M, O'Loughlin VD. How the potassium-sodium pump works. In: *Human Anatomy*. New York: McGraw-Hill; 2006. Available at: http://bit .ly/6Mwwp. Accessed September 14, 2010.

National Institute of Neurological Disorders and Stroke. NINDS multiple sclerosis information page. In: *Multiple Sclerosis: Hope Through Research*. Available at: http://www.ninds.nih.gov/disorders/multiple_sclerosis/multiple _sclerosis.htm. Accessed January 2010.

Newland PK, Naismith RT, Ullione M. The impact of pain and other symptoms on quality of life in women with relapsing-remitting multiple sclerosis. *J Neurosci Nurs*. December 2009;41(6):322–328.

Nocentini U, Tedeschi G, Migliaccio R, Dinacci D, et al. An exploration of anger phenomenology in multiple sclerosis. *Eur J Neurol*. December 2009;16(12):1312–1317.

O'Connell D. Is it an MS attack—or not? *InsideMS*. July–September 2004; 59–63. Available at: http://www.nationalmssociety.org/download.aspx?id=86. Accessed September 14, 2010.

Siegert RJ, Abemethy DA. Depression in multiple sclerosis: a review. *J Neurol, Neurosurg Psychiatry*. 2005;76(4):469–475.

Tateno A, Jorge RE, Robinson RG. Pathological laughing and crying following traumatic brain injury. *J Neuropsychiatry Clin Neurosci*. 2004;16(4): 426–434.

Trapp BD, Nave KA. Multiple sclerosis: an immune or neurodegenerative disorder? *Annu Revi Neurosci*. 2008;31:247–269.

Van der Werf SP, Evers A, Jongen PJH, Bleijenberg G. The role of helplessness as mediator between neurological disability, emotional instability, experienced fatigue and depression in patients with multiple sclerosis. *Multiple Sclerosis*. February 2003;9(1):89–94.

Weiner HL. The challenge of multiple sclerosis: how do we cure a chronic heterogeneous disease? *Ann Neurol*. March 2009;65(3):239–248.

2

The Mind–Body Connection

The mind–body connection has, in the past 30 years or so, become a subject of great interest in the medical community, as well as a source of information for those who have been served by these professionals. It is an interesting fact that, although people were seeking alternative medical intervention, many natural interventions, such as laughter, were being overlooked. The tide has now turned despite the fact that there is still a need for more, biologically based evidence to support alternatives to traditional medicine. However, laughter is now on the medical radar and its application appears to be aimed in the right, positive direction, even in the halls of medical schools. Of course, the Europeans have been using alternative therapies for many years and some of their studies are now being examined more closely to see if there are additional treatments with promise.

Prior to the acceptance of the intimate relationship between what we think and physically feel and the actual workings of our body, there was little in the way of practical intervention of a self-help nature. Self-help was pushed to the side and its use wasn't highly regarded, but that's changed, too. There are many forms of self-help and their time has come. Intense research over the past several decades not only has now shown the strength of the relationship between the mind and the body, but it also has explored the underlying biology. This connection was vital if self-help was to be seen as having a solid scientific base, and now we are beginning to get the results.

The way in which the mind interacts with the body and how the body responds is an active area of research. However, it is now becoming apparent that there is sufficient support regarding a delicate balance being maintained between the two. This balance lies at the heart of our physical and mental health. It also is responsible for helping our immune system fight disease. Not only does our mind affect how our body produces health-promoting substances, it also helps the body to reduce substances that could cause physical damage, such as the stress hormone cortisol. This hormone is the central factor in inflammation, a possible signature feature of autoimmune disorders.

Psychoneuroimmunology

In the medical community, the mind–body connection is referred to as psychoneuroimmunology (PNI). PNI has become the medical specialty that deals with the "mind–body connection," but not everyone is satisfied with describing the relationship this way.

For Dr. Stefan Gold, a neuropsychologist researcher in the multiple sclerosis (MS) program at the David Geffen School of Medicine at the University of California, Los Angeles (UCLA), the research is relatively clear that something is happening in MS that is not purely a reaction to a neurological disease that leads to high rates of depression. Looking at fatigue and depression from a patient's perspective seems to indicate that they can overlap. Even from a physician's point of view, they can overlap, but may be reflections of *two or three different underlying mechanisms*. This is where the science comes in. As Dr. Gold explained, this is an important factor. Health care providers may be treating these symptoms the same way, but they're coming from a different mechanism of underlying biology that may impede our ability to treat depression or fatigue.

Dr. Gold isn't discouraging treatment but merely indicating that we need more treatments. Care providers also need to recognize that the relationship isn't as simple as being able to effect some change in one or two neurotransmitters. The relationship is much more complex in his way of thinking.

Dr. Gold indicated that:

We're looking at symptomatic, targeted depression treatment and, in fact, there is some evidence to suggest depression is underdiagnosed in MS patients. But even if it is detected, we're trying to treat it with some treatments like psychotherapy and antidepressant medication and the efficacy depends on what we believe actually caused the depression. It looks like major depression in a psychiatric population because there are the same symptoms, but it's caused by something else. The usual pharmacologic form of treatment, such as the SSRI (selective serotonin reuptake inhibitor) medications, are not always helping because the depression is actually the result of another physical process.

As Dr. Gold sees it, it's not the usual brain neurotransmitter substances that are at the heart of the depression of patients with MS, and yet these are what the medications target. This may account for the drugs lack of efficacy in a percentage of the patients with MS. It should be noted, however, that even in persons without MS who are depressed, not all of the medications, the SSRIs and serotonin norepinephrine reuptake inhibitors (SNRIs) included, work effectively. The entire question of depression and which medications work most effectively would need to be based on something that provides a biological or medical test as a means of evaluation and there is no such guide at this time.

A diagnosis of depression, unlike much of the other medical disorders, is based solely on *symptoms*, not blood work, lumbar punctures, brain scans, or anything else. We don't even have tests to tell much about internal body changes when treated with antidepressant medications. The effort has to be trial-and-error until a medication that works *for that person* is finally found. The waiting can be draining and irritating to patients as they find themselves receiving serial trials of multiple medications without much benefit.

The question of efficacy of treatment also depends upon what some researchers have referred to as the cross-talk communication within our body's nervous system. In other words, it is a system of communication that works bidirectionally to *both promote and inhibit* a certain reaction from taking place. Therefore, there is a push-and-pull action going on at all times with the ideal state being one of balance. The actions are not necessarily entirely physical or psychological, but an inadequately understood combination of the two. However, the fact that there is a psychological component is reason for hope. If we can use our minds in bringing about change in our physical functioning, it promises to be an outstanding move in the right direction for medicine. Moreover, there is evidence that this is a very real possibility.

The immune system is slowly giving up some of its secrets. Researchers have also found that not only does the immune system protect us from disease, but they also now know that there is an additional connection that allows it to control brain activity for both sleep and body temperature. Undoubtedly there are many other areas where aspects of the immune system have a major impact on our bodies, but these have yet to be discovered.

This system even has an effect on our ability to experience appropriate moods. For that reason, we now know that many, if not all, of the autoimmune disorders such as MS, diabetes, lupus, arthritis, and others, all have a component of a mood disturbance that is, in part, caused by the immune system. Exactly how it does cause mood disturbances is still a question for researchers to answer.

The Immune System

A quick overview of the immune system indicates that several different blood components, including the five kinds of white cells, are our body's main defenders. One white blood cell class, the lymphocytes, appears to be the primary player in some of the activity in the immune system. These cells make up the group of cells that is responsible for seeking out and destroying dangerous substances in our body.

Some of this destruction involves actually killing the host cells for viruses so that the virus cannot grow inside the cell and then releasing thousands of new copies of itself into the blood. The problem arises when these white cell defenders *identify a patient's own healthy body cells* as "invaders" or, perhaps more properly, as "invaded." Then they mistakenly begin their protective action to surround the invader and an inflammatory process begins that is meant to contain and destroy this invader. There is no invader, but the process continues as though there were and the healthy cells begin to be destroyed.

All of these cells work in concert with brain and nervous system structures that are intended to be marshaled during periods of external or internal danger. An example might be when a vicious animal were running toward you in an attack. In this circumstance, your brain, sensing the danger, would immediately initiate actions that would ultimately allow you to flee or to fight.

In addition to taking actions to run away or defend yourself, the brain would begin a process that would release energy into your muscles, control your digestion, and even help your blood to clot if you were injured. This is in the presence of real danger. However, this same reaction can take place in the absence of any obvious danger, such as in a social situation where you become extremely stressed and anxious. The same fear reaction is initiated despite the absence of real physical danger. The body's nervous system and the brain begin to pour out stress hormones and prepare for defense. It's a stress reaction that's inappropriate and destructive.

The research of Hans Selye outlined this overreaction on the part of the brain and illustrated how these rogue reactions result in physical exhaustion and damage. This is a response to what is now known as the "fight or flight" phenomenon.

However, there may be an unseen confounding factor here. It may be that an unrestrained or unregulated immune response in the case of MS may be responding to *little or nothing at all.*

The problem becomes, therefore, to seek these as-yet-unknown factors. Lacking such evidence may lead to patients with MS feeling they are responsible for their own exacerbations. Just as we don't yet know the many things that initiate the MS process, we must take care not to blame the exacerbations on the person living with MS. Stress may play a major role, but it may be quite different in each person.

Researchers who are studying depression have indicated that the evidence for an inflammatory basis for depression was strong after having found higher levels of inflammatory substances in patients with depression. In fact, in treatment with interferon, up to 50% of the patients receiving it became depressed. Such evidence strengthens the basis for making a biological case for depression. It is this fact that has led to research looking at treatments for depression targeted not at neurotransmitters, which is currently the case, but at inflammatory processes.

One promising area of investigation is in the blood's cytokines, which can be inflammatory agents as well as modulators of mood and behavior. Research published by a task force of the American Academy of Neurology noted that data, first published in 2000, showed "the occurrence of stressful life events was associated with a significantly increased risk of a new . . . MRI brain lesion eight weeks later." These data were felt to be a clear indication of clinical flare-ups of MS symptoms along with evidence on neuroimaging markers of brain inflammation.

During periods of infection, there are *high concentrations of the cytokines* that cause inflammation. There exists a theory that suggests that the Epstein-Barr virus (EBV) may be at the heart of MS. This theory has been investigated further by neurologists at the Harvard School of Public Health and the Walter Reed Army Institute of Research. Their findings, based on follow-up of thousands of individuals over several years, have added to the debate about this virus being a contributory factor in the development of MS. One of the researchers, Dr. Alberto Ascherio, suggested that, "Until now, we knew that virtually all MS patients are infected with EBV."

The result of the inflammation is that there are significant changes in sleep, eating behavior, libido, social interaction, and a lowering of mood. These same symptoms form a major portion of the complex of major depressive symptoms, and this has led to something called the "sickness hypothesis." So, is it an under-the-radar illness that may be the cause of depressive flare-ups? Some would think so.

We know that extended inflammatory conditions can lead to cell death, known as *apoptosis*, with resulting functional damage. Extending this, we can see this may provide a rationale for a connection between cognitive decline and memory impairment in patients with MS where inflammation is a major issue. The waters are still murky.

Is it the stress that a person perceives, the inflammation that brings on depression that has been perceived as stress-initiated, both of these, or some variant? It's probably all that were mentioned. Yes, it's still a good idea to develop stress-coping techniques as one protective measure because there is a stress component according to current theories. However, there may also be an inflammatory component as has been indicated. Knowing what we can do about modulating the immune system through active participation in nonmedical programs brings hope in either perspective.

Helplessness

These studies clearly indicated not only the connection between stress and physical damage, but also the additional role of inflammation in feelings of depression resulting in helplessness in the face of stressful circumstances. Helplessness, of course, can be related to significant mood changes in any person with a chronic illness. Experiencing a sense of helplessness over one's illness is a mitigating stressful factor, potentially, in the course of the disease. Therefore, this would establish the use of psychotherapy in the treatment of MS as both therapeutic and helpful in creating a sense of empowerment. As we shall see, that is exactly what Dr. Gold sees as additional and useful complementary work to be done.

Helplessness was also seen in the landmark work of psychologist Dr. Martin Seligman of the University of Pennsylvania who showed that there was a direct relationship between a sense of helplessness and the development of depression. Once again, the psychological level may have initiated not only a negative mental perspective on one's ability to control one's life, but it may also have promoted an action on a biological level.

Unfortunately, Seligman's studies were confined to psychological evaluations and were never extended to physiological measures to strengthen the argument for this potential connection. For Seligman, it was a solely psychological disorder. But the work that has followed Seligman's experiments indicates there is a mechanism for certain forms of depression that lies in the body's ability to produce or inhibit substances that affect mood and the immune system's functioning.

The psychological aspects of a helplessness belief may actually initiate changes in brain chemistry geared to promote depression, so the psychological intervention directed at alleviating depression may be seen as, likewise, being able to *inhibit this biological helplessness reaction*. It's mind–body all over again.

You'll see later in this book that psychotherapy and muscle actions, such as almost any form of muscular activity including walking, according to some current research, can have definite beneficial effects on mood. Both forms of therapy appear to affect neurotransmitters responsible for mood regulation. Some researchers are indicating that it can even promote brain growth, which is one of the most exciting and promising findings recently.

Medications, which are primarily in the SSRI and SNRI groups, as we've indicated, can cause a mushroominglike effect of brain receptors as well as a retention effect of neurotransmitters between neurons, which allows chemical messengers to function more effectively. It's like giving these chemical substances more places to land on neurons and then keeping them there longer where they can do the most good. The fact that these medications do not work as well in all patients with MS, as indicated by Dr. Gold, would seem to point to an additional mechanism of depression and that appears to be a function of the immune system.

It is the opinion of Dr. Robert Sapolsky of the Stanford University School of Medicine, as it is of other researchers, that one or more of the stress hormones may play a major role in the development of depression. Dr. Sapolsky, again, stresses the complexity of the actions involved.

Cytokines are small proteins released by cells that have a specific effect on the interactions between cells. Some can trigger inflammation and respond to infection. These inflammatory cytokines have been shown to have a disturbing effect on behavior and mood. Dr. Gold spoke on the issue of these proteins and their role in inflammation:

> Some of the research has indicated that . . . [in laboratory experiments involving the injection of cytokines,] there are behaviors that indicate . . . more anxiety, less interest in exploring, and neglect of (the) young. So there is definitely something about inflammation that needs fuller investigation, especially when talking about depression as an inflammatory disease and its possible implications for MS patients.

Brain scans, Dr. Gold observed, show quite different images. "That is to say, if you get a brain scan of a person with depression, you would not see the indications that we see on brain scans with MS patients." So, although there might be some common shared mechanisms underlying depression as an inflammatory disease, it's not apparent in the brain scans of non-MS individuals. There is no distinctly apparent physical feature (such as a plaque) on a scan, whereas the patients with MS may show these features.

The Immune System and Depression

Dr. Gold continued,

> If you take an MS patient who is depressed and compare that patient to someone who is seen as psychiatrically depressed without MS, you do see some differences in some biologic systems which are usually not described in psychiatric patients. One difference is an elevated level of stress hormones, such as cortisol, and there are certain patterns regarding how that system is dysregulated. The second thing you see is damage in brain areas that are involved in mood regulation such as the hippocampus which causes memory and mood problems.

24

We have seen that chronic, stressful experiences and emotions influence how our immune system functions. Not only is there a relationship between the mind and the body, but also one where how the body reacts to physical or emotional threats and disease agents as well as *how we psychologically approach stressful events*, that are central to mood changes. Therefore, once again, the case is being made and we see that there is room in MS therapies for self-help techniques.

Dr. Gold explained both the history of PNI and his wish to call it by another and more appropriate name in his opinion. "Yes, it's a two-way street in terms of communication, surely, but I'm trying to avoid the term PNI because it has been so loosely used outside the medical community."

He prefers to change the name of PNI to neuroimmunology because he believes that PNI no longer truly expresses what is being discussed. It has been used in several different contexts in a nonmedical setting. What PNI means to Dr. Gold is the interdisciplinary science that investigates biological connections among the brain, the immune system, and the hormone system. Therefore, he indicated that if you believe that this connection truly exists, "it may be that Western medicine has lost about 200 years in terms of the mind-body model." Dr. Gold, however, doesn't believe in looking backward but forward. "Now there is a great body of evidence that there is direct communication between all of these systems. We know that, if one of these systems starts attacking, there's clearly something wrong with the communication. But what?"

It is the usual case for the immune system, the brain, and the endocrine system to form a coordinated communication network that is in balance and that direct each other. Researchers try to discover how an abnormal nonworking communication figures into neuroimmunology. In MS, they study the question of how that might be different in something like major depression. This adds a new perspective regarding where to look for those *undiscovered connections*. It is a vital clue that can advance medical knowledge, and each piece of the puzzle enlightens scientists and extends that knowledge base.

A Century of Discovery

The idea of the mind–body connection, as Dr. Gold explained, isn't a new one; it's only new in that we can now show it on a biological level with science to back up the beliefs expressed in the 19th century.

"The whole field has come full circle in that there is a pretty well-established link between experiencing periods of intense stress, and having a relapse of MS and that idea has been floating out there for a long time."

The French physician Jean-Martin Charcot first described MS in the 19th century and, as Dr. Gold indicated, he

> suspected that stress had something to do with it. He's the father of modern neurology. Nobody knew how to explain it because we didn't know enough about molecular mechanisms of stress. The work of Seyle in the 50s showed extreme stress had biological ramification, and now we have a better understanding of the mechanism of stress hormones. So, how can something that I perceive, psychologically, have biological consequences? This was the first time we had a mechanism.

Stress and the Immune System

The scientific discovery that Dr. Gold mentioned is related to the role of stress and the immune system that appeared to be contradictory in MS. Stress, it would seem, appears to increase stress hormones that *cause the immune system to ramp down*. However, in a system such as MS, where *the immune system is already overly active*, shouldn't stress be a good thing because of this action of damping down the immune system? This poses a major scientific challenge in light of current medical knowledge.

"Shouldn't that mean that stress would be good here? Again, this shows how complicated the equation is. It's a paradox in MS. We gained more and more insight into what's really going on here and now we have really good data." Some of the latest data, Dr. Gold suggested, hasn't been published yet.

He went on to discuss one particularly relevant study that wasn't designed in a laboratory but actually happened in the field. Scientists were quick to realize the use of this serendipitous consequence and set to work to begin their investigation.

> About 25 recent studies show the association between stress and MS. One study was done during the 33-day war between Lebanon and Israel and it showed that there was about a threefold increase in MS relapse. They plotted the data in four-week intervals and there was a relationship between

higher levels of military attack and self-reported higher levels of stress as well as relapse.

One thing that the people in the area could not avoid and probably felt helpless about was the bombing and the military activity. This sense of helplessness, as we now know, leads to depression that affects the immune system. As Dr. Gold points out in his interview, we now have clear evidence of this dramatic connection. Here, the helplessness is translated into exacerbations of MS.

Ten years ago, they said there really wasn't any clear evidence to make the case for stress and physical disorders. Now, we can do research where we use two groups; one in stress management and one not in stress management classes. In fact, that's a study that's going on right now. The primary outcome they will be looking at is what can be seen on MRI scans and relapse outcomes.

The question to be answered, obviously, is whether psychological interventions are effective in alleviating symptoms related to stress.

One study that Dr. Gold sees as particularly relevant to the relationship between stress and how depression and stress reactions can be treated with both psychological and pharmacologic means was done by his colleague. "One thing that was really striking, a few years ago, was a study by my colleague Dr. David Mohr which nicely demonstrates this bi-directionality."

The first thing that Mohr showed was that if you have a patient with MS who is depressed and you treat the depression, it doesn't matter whether you treat it with psychotherapy or pharmacologic intervention, *you get a decrease in inflammatory markers*. This would indicate that it is related, so *you can change the biology* and get a change in the depression, and you can do it behaviorally without medications. The result is a decrease in the depression, either way. Again, evidence is unfolding that emphasizes the effectiveness of more than one mode of treatment for MS-related depression and one of those effective treatments is behavioral therapy.

The usual explanation 20 or 30 years ago, Dr. Gold said:

Would have been, "Yeah, they're depressed but there's nothing we can do about that and it has nothing to do with the disease." They felt that it was just a reaction to the disease and that if there were something that would stop the disease, they wouldn't be depressed, anymore.

First of all, we don't have . . ., a cure for MS, but we're now beginning to understand that the actual disease may do something to the brain that leads to depression and that it isn't a psychological reaction, but a biological consequence.

Researchers have now come to see, on a basic scientific level, that it is the underlying depression that is active, and this line of thinking is receiving more credibility because of recent breakthroughs. It is becoming a hot topic in research because there are new research tools to investigate it. As Dr. Gold said, "If you have systems, and you can show how the molecular pathways are working, you can demonstrate this connection, and that's when it starts getting really interesting."

From this breakthrough, many more have followed as researchers spread an ever-widening net of interest in the area.

Exercise and Brain Function

This bidirectional finding is very hopeful because it would seem to indicate that we can affect our emotional states by what we do physically, such as exercise, laughter, biofeedback, relaxation breathing, and even creative daydreaming. This is an incredible breakthrough for the person who wonders, "but what can I do?" The number of things that can be done increases as does our knowledge of our mysterious biology.

One area receiving intense scrutiny and one in which there has been some controversy is exercise. Dr. Gold said:

"One very interesting area that is proving of great benefit is exercise. Exercise has an effect on mood. It's an antidepressant and there's a lot of scientific evidence right now that shows that it actually affects the brain directly and promotes new connections in the brain."

Exercise seems to kick-start repair mechanisms in the brain and promotes proliferation of molecules that protect neurons from damage. This evidence is based on laboratory studies, but there is some evidence that suggests that this may not only happen in laboratories, but it may apply to people living with MS, too.

The controversy around MS and exercise stems from the fact that many years ago, patients with MS were advised to avoid any exercise that raised their core body temperature, and Dr. Gold addressed this.

For the longest time, MS patients have been advised not to exercise. The thinking was that, if your core body temperature goes up, symptoms can get much worse. These are actually pseudo-exacerbations because when the body temperature comes down to normal, they disappear. It's true that MS patients do experience these exacerbations. They are not just imagining them. Patients would tell their doctors that whenever they exercised, they get worse and then the neurologist would tell them not to exercise.

In light of the new evidence, this theory no longer holds for MS and there have been several recent studies that have correlated exercise (specifically yoga) with lessening the symptoms of MS.

Also, not exercising means not getting a cardiovascular workout. Dr. Gold continued,

Now we actually have evidence that it goes the other way around; there might be a direct impact of exercise on the disease itself. Exercise can be seen as immunomodulatory and it tends to bring the immune system back down into the middle range, it affects your stress hormones, which are bad, and it has a direct effect on the brain. We don't believe anymore that it's bad for MS patients; that's been clearly established. The positive aspects that I outlined were immediately apparent in MS patients.

Dr. Gold pointed out that moderate, even really lower capacity exercise has been proved by randomized controlled studies not only to have a good effect on things like quality of life, depression, and fatigue, but may also affect walking ability. There are studies, he said, that show it may *protect the brain* and may help the brain *recover from injuries*.

"A huge literature exists that now narrows exercise benefits down to the molecular level. This is one of the big behavioral things that people can do to help themselves." The case is being made, therefore, for people to be more proactive about their disease than ever before. These new insights provide increased hope that continued effort and motivation can be two of the strongest factors working on behalf of people with MS. The one thing remaining, however, is to get this new knowledge out to *all* health care providers and those living with the disease alike.

Another researcher, Dr. Ruchika Prakash, a clinical psychologist at Ohio State University, has been studying the effects of exercise and cognition. Her research is discussed in Chapter 5.

Lifestyle Changes

Dr. Gold points out a few other things as well:

> In general, since we have the stress hormone link to all kinds of negative things, we know that stress is bad for MS. So, anything that decreases your stress is good. But, obviously, we can't tell people not to have any stressful events in their lives, but there's a possibility that, *depending on how you deal with your stressors*, it may have the potential of protecting your biology.
>
> While the potential exists that things other than exercise and stress reduction may be beneficial, there is insufficient evidence to provide definite evidence for the effectiveness, on a biological level, of other modalities MS patients may use. Neither is there any evidence to suggest that anyone brought on their disorder because they couldn't handle stress appropriately. So, labeling people with things like "Type A" personalities isn't useful or helpful when considering MS and its onset.
>
> The lack of solid evidence does not indicate, either way, that patients who do not experience benefit from things other than exercise should see themselves as responsible for their disorder's current state because of lack of effort or motivation.

Here Dr. Gold offered a cautionary note. "While patients may wish to utilize many modalities other than exercise, this may or may not result in a favorable outcome for them on an individual basis. Hope is something everyone needs to maintain, but within reasonable boundaries." Notice that Dr. Gold indicated it was *on an individual basis*, pointing to the continuing mystery of why something that works for one person may not work for another. The thing to do, if advisable, is to see if you benefit from it, but give it a decent chance of taking effect before you walk away from it. This is where continued motivation plays such an important role.

Perhaps what Dr. Gold was alluding to was that if it doesn't harm you in any way, things other than traditional approaches to MS might be worthwhile exploring, but, as the saying goes, *caveat emptor* (let the buyer beware). Also, be sure to run any nontraditional methods by your primary care physician before you engage in them.

Regarding the question of depression as part of the whole question of immune system involvement, Dr. Gold addressed it in terms of fatigue and depression. "There is some evidence that what causes the fatigue and depression may be a slightly different mechanism." The search for evidence regarding this mechanism, he said, continues; he indicated that the biology is still eluding scientists but they feel they are hot on its trail and persistence will pay off in the future.

Depression and Multiple Sclerosis

One of the things that needs to be considered is how depression is evaluated with questionnaires. These tests can have confounding factors such as assessing physical symptoms that skew the results, possibly improperly, in the direction of depression. According to Dr. Gold:

> It seems that there's a certain component of depression that can hit you at any time in your disease, and this kind of depression tends to be relatively stable.
>
> There is another type of depression that is based on physical fatigue and that type of depression seems to oscillate a bit more. The stable part seems to be associated with certain biological changes in the mood center of the brain and a change in your neuroanatomy. The fatigue type of depression is more associated with acute changes in your inflammatory system.
>
> Your symptoms are always going to be the sum of those two things, but any treatment that targets only one or the other will only affect a portion of it. This would suggest that we need different, possibly multiple strategies for treatment.

The idea that depression is caused by specific neurotransmitters alone, such as the ones currently being treated with antidepressant medications, fails to make a convincing case for Dr. Gold in terms of the newest scientific evidence. He believes that although, on average, depression may be related to changes in certain neurotransmitters such as serotonin or dopamine, on an individual level it may be very different. For that reason, he believes these medications won't work on everyone. No two people are the same. Not all types of depression are the same, and different types of depression are caused by different things and not always these two neurotransmitters.

The different responses among people remain one aspect of MS itself that still remains a question for the medical community. Dr. Gold said:

> There appears to be a similarity in MS where some people respond very well to one treatment and other people don't have the same level of response. This is even seen in the relapsing and remitting form of MS where some people will have three relapses in two years and be in a wheelchair and some people have one relapse and then nothing for 20 years. So, there has to be some variance in the disease to account for these differences. Also, some relapses are quite different with some patients having tingling in their fingers, others with vision loss and still others who are unable to get out of bed. They are all called relapses.

Although a great deal of research has been done, there is still more to be discovered and the promise of important, innovative discoveries in the future is very real. Researchers, in fact, believe that adding to this knowledge base will enable both patient and professional to work more effectively toward combating MS.

Interestingly enough, the Greek philosopher Aristotle was reported to have said, "You should not treat a body without a soul." What he was referring to was what the Roman poet Virgil referred to as "mind moves matter."

Depression Prior to Diagnosis

It was Charcot in the 19th century who made the observation that it was important to know not only what was going on in the patient's body, but also what was going on in the patient's head, as Virgil had suggested. We have now seen that even prior to a diagnosis of another possible autoimmune disorder, a significant number of patients will develop depressed mood. Patients with acquired immunodeficiency syndrome (AIDS), as well as those with upper respiratory tract infections and the elderly with urinary tract infections, also show changes in mood.

The one thing that is common in all of these patients is that they are suffering from an infection or inflammatory disorder probably caused by the immune system trying to combat the infection. So, first, we may have the disorder starting, then the mood change. Or do we? Again, here is a medical example of "which came first, the chicken or the egg?" Did the mood change occur prior to the evidence of an inflammatory process or did the inflammatory process cause the mood change?

The interesting thing is that this research points to the fact that *it is not that the person knows* they have a chronic disorder and then develops depression in response to that diagnosis. It may be just the opposite. The depression arises, as some research suggests, *prior to the diagnosis*, which means it is not a matter of the person becoming depressed because they have received the diagnosis. *It's not all in the person's mind*, but is a disorder of bodily functioning. Theoretically, the depression may act as a harbinger of an as-yet-undiagnosed inflammatory process. It's definitely a question to be explored.

This line of investigation should mean examining the medical records of a person with MS for evidence of preexisting depression. If the depression is a result of unseen inflammatory or other changes brought on by some type of abnormal physical process, it can go far to help those diagnosed with MS better cope with the depression. It could also mean a lot to those scientists looking for a cure. There is never a gain in blaming a person for his or her depression.

The fact is that depression exists in a large number of patients with MS and only a small part of it may be attributed to the initial shock of the diagnosis. This distress can be addressed with cognitive therapy and, as we've seen, exercise. Both of these modalities help that all-important mind–body connection because depression is both physical and a mental adjustment.

Remember, it's an adjustment and adjustments can be dealt with. Dealing with the depression on this level can tap into that all-important feedback circuit in our immune system that can contribute to more efficient immune functioning. In that way, therapy and exercise may do more than help with the depression; they may, in some small way, be reparative, as we've seen from the research Dr. Gold discussed in this chapter.

Medical experts are hopeful that this new perspective can provide some reassurance to people living with MS that they can, indeed, make a difference in their own health by employing self-help strategies. We'll deal with these in later chapters.

Further Reading

American Psychological Association. Mind/body health: the effects of traumatic stress. Available at: http://www.apas.org/helpcenter/stress.aspx. Accessed December 2009.

Anisman H, Merali Z. Cytokines, stress, and depressive illness. *Brain Behav Immun*. 2002;16(5):513–524.

Axtell RC, de Jong BA, Boniface K, et al. T helper type 1 and 17 cells determine efficacy of interferon-β in multiple sclerosis and experimental encephalomyelitis. *Nat Med* [serial online]. March 28, 2010. Available at: http://www.msrc.co.uk/downloads/MS2K.pdf. Accessed September 14, 2010.

Dantzer R, O'Connor JC, Freund GG, Johnson RW, Kelley, KW. From inflammation to sickness and depression: when the immune system subjugates the brain. *Nat Rev Neurosci*. 2008;9(1):46–56.

Goldberger L, Breznitz S, eds. *Handbook of Stress: Theoretical and Clinical Aspects*. New York: The Free Press; 1982.

Irwin MR, Miller AH. Depressive disorders and immunity: 20 years of progress and discovery. *Brain Behav Immun*. 2007;21(4):374–383.

Kern S, Ziemssen T. Brain-immune communication psychoneuroimmunology of multiple sclerosis. *Mult Scler* [serial online]. September 19, 2007. Available at: http://82.194.73.155/~lxmemrgb/attachments/026_ELA_anexo_IV.pdf. Accessed September 15, 2010.

Leonard BE, Myint A. The psychoneuroimmunology of depression. *Hum Psychopharmacol*. 2009;24(3):165–175.

McCain NL, Gray DP, Walter JM, Robins, J. Implementing a comprehensive approach to the study of health dynamics using the psychoneuroimmunology paradigm. *ANS Adv Nurs Sci*. 2005;28(4):320–332.

McFarland HF, Martin R. Multiple sclerosis: a complicated picture of autoimmunity. *Nat Immunol*. 2007;8(9):913–919.

ScienceDaily. Further evidence links Epstein-Barr virus and risk of multiple sclerosis. March 5, 2010. Available at: http://www.sciencedaily.com/releases/2010/03/100304165900.htm#. Accessed April 2010.

Sospedra M, Martin R. Immunology of multiple sclerosis. *Annu Rev Immunol*, 2005;23:683–747.

Watkins A. *Mind-Body Medicine: A Clinician's Guide to Psychoneuroimmunology*. New York: Churchill Livingstone; 1997.

Ziemssen T, Kern S. Psychoneuroimmunology—cross-talk between the immune and nervous systems. *J Neurol*. 2007;254(suppl 2):118–111.

3

Riding the Rollercoaster of Multiple Sclerosis

Multiple sclerosis's waxing-and-waning symptom pattern may cause people with MS to experience mood turmoil on a daily, weekly, or monthly basis. It's been described as an emotional rollercoaster by some patients.

When faced with this emotional turmoil, patients planning future activities, making career choices or changes, deciding on family matters, and even thinking about retirement can find themselves in an uncertain world that calls for day-to-day tweaks or taxing adjustments. Persons with MS can have a sense of not knowing what tomorrow will bring, because they have no way of predicting these mood changes. It can seem, at times, like a hopeless task dealing with the mood shifts, the anxiety, the pain, the sleep disturbance, and the fatigue.

The situation can result in a feeling of loss of control and unwanted dependence, and a possible dilemma of being lost in your own life. In addition, it is the not-knowing aspect that increases any physical and mental stress you may feel. It can seem like a resistant, uncharted trek in a no-man's land, exploring a territory without ever knowing what pitfalls may lie ahead. This, of course, is where education plays a highly important role.

Acquiring knowledge about your disorder, its possible symptoms, and the means to treat it are all vital factors in your continued health. The saying "Knowledge is power" is quite relevant here because knowledge also provides a sense of handling stress, which is magnified when something is "unknown" as much about MS can be.

Knowledge of how MS arises, what it involves, and what the future may hold in terms of research can increase the sense of control and decrease a portion of this stress. A future-oriented, positive perspective, therefore, is highly desirable. It may be as beneficial in terms of the progression of MS, according to some experts, as treatments offered by health care professionals.

There can still be unpredictable changes in mood or a chronic sense of a low mood, however. How does anyone cope when constantly faced, as the person with MS is, with sudden shifting moods, periods of depression, and an inability to effectively cope in the face of these moods? It can be a disappointing time, and it is a time that requires great fortitude in the face of poorly understood biological forces. The enemy seems relentless. How do you, in fact, fight an enemy you cannot see and over which you feel you have little or no control? It's an enemy that saps your motivation and your energy. How can you fight when you find yourself so drained? You take action even when you feel you can't and that's where the idea of resilience comes to bear.

Resilience and Illness

The concept of resilience has become one in which many psychologists have shown great interest. Some researchers have called it the ability to thrive in the face of adversity, and they have even proposed that adversity can bring about benefits for these thrivers. They see it as promoting abilities that were there, but were never called to action.

In one instance, the researcher compared it to a child who developed one of those all-too-common childhood illnesses and who, after overcoming the illness, has immunity as a result. So, too, coming out of the throes of a psychological trauma, as a result of medical illness, can support new strategies and encourage growth. Call it "stress inoculation" if you wish because that may well be what you're doing.

The stressor of a medical illness can be a threat or a loss, but the sense of it being an emerging challenge that must be met can materialize. Thriving, and its attendant resilience, is meeting this challenge rather than succumbing to the threat and exhibiting a sense of helplessness. In MS, where relapses may be occurring, it can be likened to a form of desensitization where you meet each relapse, overcome it, and you go on with your life. Each event is viewed through the lens of prior successes and the threat is lessened.

This pattern of relapse and reemergence to activity places the relapse in a new context, one where MS patients have an opportunity to appreciate their ability to recover and to bounce back, albeit slowly. You'll read about examples of patients who have done just that in later chapters.

Rather than forming a negative view of a relapse, it is possible to build on prior episodes and become even more effective. The skills you acquire by going through these relapses need to be appreciated and acknowledged for what they are and what they do for you. Too often there may be the tendency to downplay these accomplishments, which is counterproductive. Beating yourself up never helped any situation, especially where this type of stress may do more harm than anything else. Be an effective coach for yourself and you'll do much better.

Just as you need to manage your external world, so, too, do you need to manage your internal world. This internal world, of course, is your emotional world and this, although unseen, plays a prominent role in your success at anything. You do this by resisting the inclination to note only major events in your life when you should be noting the value of *all events where you've succeeded in something*. Remember, skill doesn't always mean an ability to do something physically; it can also mean adding to your knowledge base so that you are mentally more effective in the future. This knowledge can lead, in the future, to an enhanced expectation of surviving any adversity that comes to you. Recall the phrase, "self-fulfilling prophecies"? It doesn't always have to mean something negative. *You can also anticipate successes.*

Therefore, to thrive requires a new mental reorganization that you may not have thought about before. How you approach something requires preparation in thinking about what you did in the past and what others have done. Put it all together and you can find a way through the maze that presents itself to you. *You don't have to reinvent the wheel*, but you have to see what others have done in similar situations and adapt it to your situation. This is your time of transformation.

An eminent psychologist, Dr. George Bonanno, a psychology department chair at Columbia University, has spent most of his career studying grief, not resilience per se, but he does see that resilience is a major factor in the grief experience.

Chronic medical illness has been seen by psychologists as having a component of grief because of the loss felt by patients. In his work, Dr. Bonanno has come to question the accepted Western notion of grief and loss and how people are expected to adjust to this loss. He, in fact, offers some interesting new insights.

People don't necessarily go through the stages of grief that have been thought of as standard, and Dr. Bonanno feels that, for each person, there is a highly personal adjustment to loss. Those who understand this and who can make the necessary adjustments possess the survival tool known as *resilience*. So, what is resilience and how do you know if you have it or don't have it, or how can you work on cultivating it?

Researchers who have studied this protective resilience factor view it on the personal or individual level as having the following factors:

- a sense of confidence in your problem-solving skills
- a strong sense of religion, spirituality, or some connection or belief of this type
- a strong social support network of family and friends

Of all three factors, social support appears to play a central and vital role in maintaining a sense of resilience in anyone with a chronic illness, according to this research. Interestingly, the research also points out that caregivers of anyone with a chronic disorder were positively affected by social support, which they indicated "contributes . . . a valuable, protective resource that enhances resilience. . . ." Accordingly, both a person with MS and anyone caring for the person can realize important benefits from their surrounding social support system. The researchers further noted that, quoting research from Masten (2001), "When adversity is relieved and basic human needs are restored, then resilience has a chance to emerge. Rekindling hope may be an important spark for the resilience processes to begin their restorative work."

Resilience, therefore, appears to be highly dependent upon revitalizing a personal sense of hope. It is this belief that contributes to the manner in which anyone meets the challenges and the changes in their life. It's not only what you do and how you cope with your illness, but also how others see you, and it helps you to maintain your sense of self and security in your own abilities.

The social network provides more than an opportunity to enjoy a laugh or offer a willing ear when you need to vent; it is "medication" for the mind and the body. Our need for nurture doesn't stop after childhood, but continues throughout our lives and it is satisfied through our being supported in more emotional, nonphysical ways than when we were children. The balm of friendship and familial attachment provides more than any prescription medication could. Most of us don't need research to tell us that, but it's good to know that cold, unsentimental science supports that belief, too.

The whole concept of resilience and social support was discussed by Dr. Bonanno when he described *durable adults* as people who went on with their lives despite unbelievable tragedy. What did they have that made this possible? He noted, when presenting information on the survivors of the Hiroshima bombings, that they had obvious, overt support from their friends, families, and neighbors. In other cases, there was a shift from making a tragedy the central focus of life to placing it in the context of one's entire life and not seeing it as an outstanding, single defining moment.

Some people, with many expected negative incidents, who participated in a study with a large urban sample appeared to have forgotten major negative occurrences, almost as though they hadn't existed. They had to be prompted to recall these events after initially indicating they had none to report. Not a sign of pathology but of perspective in a forward-looking view of their lives, this provided energy for life rather than for grieving for "what might have been." If we were going to say anything about the content of this study that would be valuable to you right now, it would be that *perspective is everything.*

Even in cases where people may have been expected to develop serious, psychiatric disorders such as posttraumatic stress disorder (PTSD), the incidents in this study had faded and some researchers believe that, rather than reliving the trauma, it may be more beneficial to focus on the current possibilities of life. The maintenance of such a here-and-now focus was seen as much more helpful in dealing with their present life situation. This perspective, the researchers indicated, serves as a *buffering effect and helps ward off both negative emotions and physical downturns.* Four components of this mindset were determination, perseverance, tenacity, and a sense of control in the face of chronic illness.

The people with MS interviewed for this book maintained this here-and-now focus with a future orientation and all of them preferred to work toward what they could do rather than what they couldn't do and what might have existed previously. Their attitudes were more self-accepting, situation specific, and solution oriented. It was "What can I do now?" rather than "What was I able to do before I was diagnosed?"

Some of them had found solutions on their own, whereas others picked up information and used it in their own lives, in their own way. They had no idea about the protective factor of such a view; they just knew it helped them to deal with each day as it came. It was a means of maintaining hope in the face of adversity.

The idea that hope may vary with daily fluctuations in emotion has to be accounted for considering that an illness such as MS affects mood in an unpredictable pattern. Hope is something that may be difficult to maintain all the time under these circumstances, but as one man said, "I may have felt bad one day, but I don't feel bad all the time, every day." He had helped himself to turn it around so that he was in the driver's seat regarding his outlook on life, not his MS-generated mood shifts. Such a new, revised orientation toward emotion, he found, was fully warranted in his case and, he believed, in the life of every person living with MS.

This man faced exacerbations of his illness with the view that he would begin to work, once more, toward regaining what he has accomplished with his treatments and his self-help exercise program. This man serves as an inspiration to all around him and he gladly shares his personal experiences so that he can help others. *Obstacles are things to be met with creativity*, as he sees it, and he shows that by meeting every one of them in ways he may never have thought he could. Each move brings him greater realization about his abilities and what he can do now.

The time had come for this man to discontinue his emotion-focused approach to life and one event brought this out clearly to him. The mood swings and irritability had come on slowly and built up when, one day, it hit the boiling point and he, in total anger and exercising the poor judgment that MS can bring, told his wife to leave. He had been married for many years and now in the blink of an eye, over something truly trivial, he wanted her to leave their home. His wife was able to step back from her husband's anger and offer reassuring words. This man's wife understood what he was experiencing and she knew that reason had to be prudently used here. It stopped him in his tracks as he realized what he was demanding. The incident helped bring on the change he needed and it made him more introspective about his past and future actions. It had been a shocking realization, and something he would have greatly regretted if she had complied with his demands. Fortunately, she understood how MS was clouding his judgment at that point.

He saw that "absolutes" got him nowhere and, like politics, he realized that *it's the power of the possible that counts*. Turning his thinking around in this way helped him get started in a healthier mental direction in his life and he steadfastly practices this each day.

Resilience and developing this perspective shouldn't be seen as the exclusive domain of people with MS; it needs to be included in the lives of those who care for them. Because stress can bring on problems in physical health and mood, it makes sense that anyone in an extremely stressful, unpredictable situation is prone to negative outcomes.

Caregivers and families need to be included in this resilience-building approach and everything in this book can be used for the benefit of persons with MS and those who love and care for them, as well. Share what you learn and you will be giving a special gift to them.

Too often, caregivers show a concern that there will be a lack of empathy for them if they attempt to get support from others. It's as though they feel they are expected to continue in silence and not to share their struggles with anyone else because that person may not understand or they will think poorly of them. Keeping their stress to themselves and not allowing others to provide the social support that is vital to anyone involved with a person with a chronic medical condition is counterproductive to any caregiver's health.

Begin the conversation. There's nothing wrong with seeking help when you need it and no one said you had to be the modern-day version of the Greek mythological Sisyphus who, for eternity, had to keep pushing a boulder up a mountainside only to have it fall back at the top.

One man looked to see what he could do for those around him who were also contending with a loved one who had MS. He felt that when he did something positive for them, it had the same effect on him and his spouse.

He wasn't a biologist, but he knew as we do that the immune system is bidirectional. Do good, receive good in return. Not selfish, but truly self-help in an application that rewards everyone. For him, it was more than working with the coordinated team of MS specialists, and it was something he could do outside the treatment plan that would increase his sense of self-esteem and empowerment.

Resilience-Building Behaviors

Not everyone is going to feel resilient after they've been given a diagnosis of a chronic medical illness. There are things, however, that have been proposed to help *develop this quality* of resilience. Looking at the steps toward resilience, we see that psychologists suggest the following:

- actively join groups such as civic, faith-based, local support groups
- see the possible rather than the catastrophic in problems you face
- accept that everything can and will change throughout life
- set realistic goals and do things on a regular basis to achieve them in any small way you can each day
- actively engage rather than detach by taking steps to combat negative stress
- initiate a search for self-discovery and personal growth
- cultivate a positive view of yourself rather than a diminished self-view
- maintain a healthy perspective on the present and the future
- work toward maintaining your sense of optimism even when you're down
- remember your needs and feelings and *be good to yourself*
- find something that enriches an aspect of your life

Use these points as guideposts or stress buffers, not absolutes. You may find that all of them can be incorporated into your life in some way but some may be a better fit now than others. When the time is right for you, you can initiate innovations into this cycle of resilience. Modify, engage, and be prepared for change and good things will lie where you may never have thought to look for them. An Eastern Indian proverb says, "*What the mind does not know, the eye does not see.*" Open your mind to possibilities and you will open your eyes to future promise.

As one woman pointed out to me, she and her family wouldn't have known such a sense of community and wouldn't have had an opportunity to experience how kind and generous others could be if it weren't for her diagnosis of MS. She saw it as something good that had come out of a problematic medical challenge and she saw that her entire family benefitted from it.

Now, she also saw how her children were incorporating the values of helping others because of their education through MS-organized activities. Her children knew the realities of the illness and saw how it could affect people in multidimensional ways. They had further evidence that it could affect their mother in many of these same functions. It was a life lesson that they learned early in their lives, not later on in adulthood.

There was no downside to her way of thinking. She knew there would probably be flare-ups of her MS, but there was a plan in place to deal with this. Her "support team" in her community was ready and willing to help as was her extended family.

One thing that she had learned was to build on her successes, not to overemphasize the negatives in her life, and to add to her arsenal of things to do to cope. The inconsistency of her symptoms was all factored into that plan.

The Four Phases of Acceptance

The idea of phases for chronic illness, rather than stages, indicates that there is a progression and a regression on the psychological and, in the case of MS patients, the medical front. Each phase also brings with it an attempt by the individual to deal with the illness or some aspect of it as it applies to his or her life. The phases that have been proposed include the following:

1. **Crisis:** In this phase, the patient is seeking relief from the psychological turmoil of having received a diagnosis of a chronic illness. He or she may look to health practitioners, various treatments, spiritual help, or even substance abuse. It is a time of intensely seeking relief from this diagnosis. It is also a time of trying to deny a diagnosis of MS, to somehow escape from it, and of hoping that a mistake has been made.

   MS can be particularly difficult to diagnose because, as has been outlined, the symptoms may not be constant. This inconsistency can lead to a belief that the diagnosis isn't "real" and weeks, months, or even years may pass before an accurate diagnosis is made. The result is that the patient feels, therefore, that valuable time may have been lost because of this lack of accurate, early diagnosis. It can mean a time of anger and of depression.

The lack of a definitive diagnosis can also increase the anxiety of a person with MS as a result. Anxiety, of course, also means that there is an increase in the individual's stress level, which engages a negative feedback loop, which can have a negative impact on health. *The vicious cycle is driven by the engine of anxiety.*

There can be disbelief regarding the accuracy of the diagnosis, a rejection of it, and even a sense of revulsion as though the body had done something horrible to the person. There may also be a sense of a loss of worth, of shame, and of noticeable disturbing attitudes expressed by family, friends, and others. Because no one knows what causes MS, the question on many people's minds may be whether it is contagious. It is, undoubtedly, a very disturbing and upsetting time in the person's life. For the person living with the disease, the primary task here is to deal with all of these factors and come to some sense that they will be able to function despite the diagnosis. It can, however, be a great struggle. Social support is vital.

2. **Stabilization:** This is a phase of becoming more familiar with the symptoms of MS and attempting to continue to lead a more or less normal life as had been led prior to the diagnosis. When the illness is stabilized and the person has achieved some sense of mental stability regarding the illness, there can be a belief that there will be no change or very little change in that person's life. This thought can cause people to fail to recognize that changes must be made to resume normal activities. It is a time that calls for pragmatism, yet it is the time that, in some sense, may be characterized by denial. Recognizing the true nature of the illness, the changes needed, and how to best plan a life around these changes are what are needed during this phase. *Denial is the enemy.*

3. **Resolution:** This is a period where acceptance, not only of the fluctuating symptoms of MS, but also of the responses of those around the person with MS is experienced. The person with MS must now face the sometimes daunting task of

attempting to construct not only a new life that now includes the illness as part of it, but also one that indicates there will probably be no return to the prior level of functioning. There can be a sense of loss for this perceived inability to return to the prior existence.

4. **Integration:** Here the individual begins to make meaningful changes not only in daily functioning, but also in his or her work life, social life, and social networks, and begins to make medical treatments and the illness a part of his or her life. It can be an extremely productive time, and even an exciting one, if seen in a positive light. The individual must remember, however, that although he or she has MS, the disorder does not define the individual as a person. The individual is still the person he or she always was, but with abilities that may be somewhat changed or limited.

   The task here is one of making acceptable choices, and those that can be handled within the context of the person's curtailed abilities. The range of possibilities must be explored, and, often, health care professionals can play an extremely useful role here. The support of family, friends, and the work environment also plays a powerful role in this phase. Everything must be carefully assessed to maximize any resources that may be helpful to the individual. As one person said, "I have MS. Now what?"

How long each phase may last is strictly individual. Medical and/or mental health professionals may put a timeframe on some of these phases, but these should be seen strictly as rather loose estimations. Whatever time you need in each of these phases to effectively pass through that phase is what will be normal for you. It is as Dr. Bonanno indicated in his research on resilience and grief; *each person in their own way, in their own time.*

Just as a normal blood pressure is really not 120/80, but some variation around those numbers, any adjustments you make to major changes in your life will be those that are practical and acceptable for you at that moment. Some people will take longer in each phase; others may go through them more rapidly. This is not a race or in any way a measure of your ability or value as a person. Viewing it as either would be a self-defeating exercise.

Of course, one aspect of the grieving process may have to do with helping others understand what you are experiencing. One woman, who had her diagnosis for over a decade, when speaking to her physician, was told, "But you look good." It angered her and she told him that it wasn't a matter of how she looked, but how she felt and she didn't feel good at all.

Months later, there was some sense of realization on his part as he told her that he had a recently discovered back problem and that now he was always in pain. "But you look so good," she told him with a smile and he answered, "Touché."

The point had been made. Both were experiencing an internal sense of pain and depression but, to look at either of them, they looked fine. If they hadn't revealed their inner pain, no one would have known, so the grief of chronic illness is very much an internal encounter with an unseen force.

Sarah, a Young Career Woman

Sarah is a young businesswoman working in a major U.S. city. She was in good health, active in various endeavors, and looking forward to a relatively uneventful but positive future. The thought never occurred to her that she would have MS at any point in her life. However, it has been less than 1 year since she received the definitive diagnosis via a spinal tap.

"I literally woke up one morning and could not see out of my left eye. It seemed very cloudy, as though I had looked into the sun, and I had blind spots. I had been having migraines and had been coming off a very stressful business week, so I thought it was a result of all of that. I took some medication for my migraine and just proceeded to go to work and ignore it because I felt I was just stressed out. I thought I would get some more sleep over the weekend and things would be fine."

Four days later, Sarah still had the problem with her vision and decided she needed to do something, so she called a 24-hour nurse help line for some assistance. "I figured it was time to reach out and see if I could find out what this was."

The nurse who was on call directed her to an area hospital that accepted walk-in patients. Sarah went to the walk-in office, fully expecting "that it would be nothing." She felt there should be no problems, and "I was in a really good place in my life." It wasn't long before the physician decided they needed one more test to make the diagnosis. "In fact, I didn't have to wait for a long time for the diagnosis, and I got it pretty quick. The worst time is the waiting and not knowing."

This was where Sarah's personal rollercoaster ride began. A portion of the ride would be precipitated by medications, which they gave her initially, prior to her spinal tap. These were anti-inflammatory steroidal medications, which caused mood swings and other problems.

Effective planning had always been part of Sarah's life and now she had to plan to handle her diagnosis and everything that might come with it. "At first, all I could think of were those pictures of people in wheelchairs, and it was a bit overwhelming. However, I decided to put my network in place so that I would be prepared for anything that might happen in the future. You have to be smart and really begin to make plans. So, for me, it's about finding out about services now so that they'll be there if and when I need them."

Deciding to handle her diagnosis in much the same manner as she would a professional project, Sarah sat down to plot out what she would do next. "I'm a pretty strong individual, but I think my family had a hard time with it. They lived far away from me. And, in some ways, that was good, because I had time to adjust and to help them adjust.

"I started out by working on a whole spreadsheet, which listed all of the doctors who were specialists in MS and the medications and the side effects. I kept the list of different neurologists, and who had recommended them and also kept recommendations from anyone who either had MS or knew someone who had MS and had received treatment. I did all my research and went through it methodically and started writing everything up, to decide with whom I should consult.

"So it's really on the patient to be active in this. It was very overwhelming and a lot of work, and sometimes you don't want to deal with it and you'd like to push it away, but that would have been a mistake.

"My family wanted to be there for me, but it was very difficult because of the distance between us. Therefore, we were trying to arrange time off from work for them and for me so that I could go for my testing. There was also a consideration of time off. My mother wanted to be with me when I went to the hospital for the tests, and she was able to be there and it was very helpful. I can understand why it would be important for someone to have this kind of support."

Not only did Sarah have to help herself remain focused and control her anxiety, but she also had to help her relatives deal with this new dilemma. "The hardest thing is that you want to put up a strong front and tell yourself it's not that bad. But when I did get the final results, I had a pretty rough day. I had thought that it wouldn't be me and that it would be okay. I thought I didn't have any other symptoms. So, maybe, I thought, it would be fine, and this was just a fluke. But then I got the results and realized that I had MS."

Seeing the diagnosis as a wake-up call was the way Sarah decided to handle it. Viewing it from this perspective, she felt, was a good thing because life change was needed. She would later receive an additional diagnosis of stress-induced asthma. "So I went from being someone who had never been in the hospital and with no medical problems to having two things, one after another, with which I had to contend. I felt my body was saying that I couldn't do what I had been doing before and that I had to make some changes."

The Internet has been one of Sarah's most valuable resources, in her opinion. "I think we're blessed with the Internet today because everyone can empower themselves with all the information out there. Unfortunately, not everyone realizes the power of the computer and its information-retrieval abilities. I've attended groups where people seem to be asking such basic questions about MS that I felt they were not going out seeking the information for themselves."

Not meaning to sound negative about others, she said, "I guess that's a way of trying to avoid making MS real for themselves. I was a little surprised to hear people saying how difficult it was to have MS." Then she realized that there were very real relevant factors that hadn't been on her radar. "Some of the things they discussed I had never considered before. So in this way, some of the groups were eye openers for me."

An issue that came up at an MS group meeting hit particularly hard and added yet another consideration to Sarah's thoughts about herself and her future. "One of the groups dealt with dating and it was especially eye opening. I thought that if this (relationship) doesn't work, I'm going to be out there dating again, so that was scary, but it was good because they walk you through a lot of situations and give you pretty concrete ways to deal with things." Sarah is in a relationship and has a very supportive boyfriend who has attended groups with her.

The question of sharing whether she had MS was something that Sarah found not too difficult, unlike a young professional man in one of the groups she attended. "There was a guy who had MS for 10 years," she said, "and this was his first meeting."

The man was a professional, young, and in a very demanding field. He had hidden his MS so well that he didn't even date because it might have opened up that conversation. Only recently, when his job required that he work extremely long hours, which sapped his strength greatly, did he have to indicate to his company that he did have MS and required some accommodation. Sarah thought, "Oh, gosh, it took him 10 years!" Therefore, for some people, it takes a long time to talk about it and a long time before they allow themselves to reach out for help.

"I've been pretty open with it, but that's just the way I am. Some people are surprised at how open I am, but occasionally, you're in a situation where the subject just comes up. For instance, I was in an exercise class that I hadn't taken before, because I had switched from another class to this one. Someone commented on a piece of equipment I was using. Then I had to explain that I was no longer in the other class because I had MS and it could have exacerbated my symptoms. She'd asked me this while I was in a crowded elevator. So I just said, 'Well, I was recently diagnosed with MS,' and then there was absolute silence in the elevator."

Stigma remains one of the problems for anyone with MS, as Sarah indicated. "A lot of people don't want to share it with anyone. They especially don't share it in the workplace. They clam up, and some people freeze up when they find out you have it. They don't want to talk about it; they don't want to deal with it. So when you share it with someone, even with your close friends or acquaintances, you don't know what reaction you're going to get until the situation is presented. I don't think anyone really knows how they might deal with the situation until it comes up." The MS groups, however, do try to prepare members for these types of situations and, for that, Sarah has been grateful.

For now, Sarah has everything in place for the future. Her MS is stabilized; she takes daily injectable medication and has had few problems with side effects. In fact, she had chosen her medication, in consultation with her neurologist, to ensure that there would be no problems in the future because she intends to have a family. "I didn't want to begin to take something that would prevent my having a family or that would present additional problems for me. I looked at the classes of medications that were available, looked at the side effects for each, and picked the one that fit my needs best."

Regarding depression, Sarah indicated that there was a family history of depression and that she had been on medication for depression for several years, so any depression associated with her MS may have been canceled out.

Two things that Sarah believes that are vital for MS patients are compliance with treatment and exercise. "I'm very involved in yoga because I find that very helpful." However, there are even a lot of equestrian programs that have been shown to be helpful in alleviating symptoms. Many of the MS chapters will have programs on site, and there are books for yoga that have modified exercises even for people in wheelchairs.

Offering some helpful suggestions, she continued, "You can always modify yoga. It starts with breathing, which helps to calm you down, gives you more oxygen, and improves your mood. You can even do it in your own home, but if you can get out to a yoga class, the social aspect can be very helpful. It's always harder to motivate yourself, if you're trying to exercise alone."

Anna, a Homemaker/Senior Citizen

Anna's MS journey is quite different from Sarah's. Rather than receiving a diagnosis quickly, Anna had to wait over two decades because of the unusual nature of her symptoms. As she tells it, "I was in college at the time, and one day, I just woke up and had a heavy feeling from the waist down. My legs felt like somebody had tied cement blocks to them. I went to the college infirmary, where the doctor asked if I were having boyfriend trouble. I told him I didn't have a boyfriend at the time and *it wasn't in my head*, it was in my legs."

When it came time to go home for the semester, Anna went to see her family doctor, who promptly put her into the hospital. "They tested me and the only conclusion that they could come to was that it was an inflammation of the spinal cord. I had two neurologists taking care of me and the symptoms just went away. But they would come back again with the change of seasons and that's the way it was until I was 45, and I started going through menopause. At that time, I was diagnosed with MS. So, I was 21 at the time I first had the leg symptoms and I was 45 when the symptoms no longer went into remission. I went to a local neurologist, who did some tests and decided that I had MS."

Anna doesn't take medication for her MS because, as she said, "When they would tell me about the side effects, I would tell them to forget it. My neurologist was very upset with me because he said that this could help me. I said to him, 'If you can find something that will reverse this and the damage that has already been done, I'll give it a try.' I really began to worry about all the other things that might happen if I took the medication, so I told them I wouldn't take it. So I don't.'"

It's been about 8 years since Anna last saw a neurologist who, at that time, ordered a magnetic resonance imaging (MRI), which indicated there were no new changes in her brain. The result seemed to provide additional evidence for Anna that she needed neither treatment from a neurologist nor medication for her MS, so she never returned.

Basically a healthy woman, Anna has no other illnesses to speak of and said, "My symptoms are really balance problems and I have to use a walker and sometimes I have problems with my bladder. I had two episodes with my eyes, however. One night I was reading in bed and it was like there was a projector in my head and it was going very fast. It lasted for about 5 minutes and then went away. Ever since that time, it's never come back."

"One other time, though, I thought I might have had a bad cold or something, because while I was lying in bed, I could feel my body tumbling as though I were dizzy and I had to hang on to the side of the bed. It lasted for a very short time and then it went away." Other than the one instance with eye problems and the feeling of dizziness while in bed, Anna has indicated that her MS is stabilized, but she does have some memory problems.

Her main problems, however, have been with her legs and her balance. "I began to feel that I was bumping into things and losing my balance, so I first used a cane and then I had to use two canes. Now I use a walker and a wheelchair for long distances."

A woman who prides herself in her ability to handle even this illness, Anna indicated, "I get very frustrated, rather than anxious or depressed, because I can't do the things I want to. It's really that the body won't let me and it's the weirdest thing because I've never had any symptoms above the waist. My weakness is all from the waist down. My arms are still okay." She has decided that she's not going to let this illness get her down, however.

Confined pretty much to her home, Anna manages to exercise on a stationary bike she keeps there. "I know I can't do that much exercise, but I try to do what I can. Of course the legs don't move the way they used to anymore, so I grab my pants and make the legs work that way. I'm trying to remain as active as I can."

One pleasure that she still enjoys is reading. "I read a lot. I don't watch television that often because I love to read and I am constantly reading books. I also do puzzles, but not as much as I could."

The fact that her legs are affected by her MS has prevented Anna from socializing as much as she might like. Therefore, once a month, she and her girlfriends get together for coffee, and it's then that she has an opportunity to express some of her feelings about her MS. "Most people don't have any clue about how difficult it is for me," she said, "but my girlfriends really seem to understand. When I talk to them, it's easier for them to understand than it is for other people. They understand my frustration with wanting to do things and not being able to and to have to wait for others to help me."

Shopping trips also present unique problems for Anna, even though she has a handicap sticker for the family car. "Do you have any idea how far away from the store entrances they've placed handicap parking at the mall? If it's a rainy day, you'll be soaked by the time you get to the door and if you're someone who has problems walking, you wouldn't want to park that far away from the store entrances." It seems that although mall designers put handicap parking into the plan, they were, like so many others, unaware of the difficulties of people who have problems walking. "Unless you experience it yourself," she said, "you really don't understand the difficulty."

"It's especially frustrating around the holidays when I want to do things in my home such as decorating or cooking and I have to wait for help to get it done. What I have to understand is that it's not at my convenience, but theirs and that's the way it seems to be. They tell me not to worry about it, but I'm concerned and it's not very helpful."

Although she didn't say it, it was obvious that Anna has to exercise quite a bit of patience not only with her body and her disability, but with having to ask for help from others and then having to wait for it. She takes it all in good humor, however, and appears to have more than a little bit of understanding of others. This may be one of her most effective coping mechanisms. Perhaps it's the quality that first led her to study health care as a young woman and which now has proven to be working in her best interests. It's never easy, however, for a "helper" to ask for help.

When talking about her energy level, Anna admits that it's in the late afternoon, just when she has to begin preparing dinner, that she is at her lowest point. "It's my legs," she said.

Despite her problems with her legs and her energy level, Anna would like to be more independent, even if she were totally in a wheelchair. The problem, as she sees it, is that wheelchairs are too cumbersome, too heavy, and don't permit the freedom that someone might want to exercise. "I'd like a smaller, lighter chair that would allow me to maneuver myself. The light chairs that they have now don't allow you to move; you need someone pushing you. Also, I'd like to go to the beach, but I can't because a wheelchair gets stuck in the sand."

Her desire to be involved in life and to enjoy it as much as possible is apparent from how she talks about accepting MS and remaining hopeful about the future. And she enjoys socializing with her friends, reading, using her pool, and going to the beach. Not once during our conversation did she complain about her illness or about her plight. She maintained an upbeat, positive attitude. If she had one wish, she'd like a wheelchair that can go over the sand at the beach, but the only one designed for that activity costs an estimated $30,000. "Who could afford that?" she asked.

William, a Mid-career Professional

William was a professional with his own firm and made the difficult decision to retire once he realized how MS was affecting his work performance. "The bad news was enough to deal with, and I thought that this was the end, not only of life as I knew it, with my wife, our young child, and the one child we were expecting, but I thought I didn't know what to expect. I didn't know how this all happened so fast and I didn't know where it would lead.

"For me, it was like an airplane experiencing really bad turbulence. You're not in control, you're not in the cockpit, you don't see the instruments. It's really what's going on in your brain. You don't know how bad this is, you don't know whether this is it when people start screaming, or it's just going to be a horrible ride. It's as though your life were going to be cut off much sooner. In an airplane, maybe you have some time to plan, but it's disconcerting.

"Then you see the look when you share it with your spouse or your immediate family. You see it on their faces and they look all poker faced. Or it's terror on their faces because, as little as you may know, you're experiencing it and they know even less. They begin to imagine the worst possible diagnosis with MS, and it's common to imagine the worst even if it may not be a reality. But that's where the mind takes over and the information in the booklets and everything else is left alone. The anxiety and the fear are almost paralyzing.

"I transferred to a second neurologist once the cognitive part started to settle in. I don't want you to think that I was doctor shopping or anything. It just seemed to make sense for me to see her and hear what I needed to do, not that I wanted to be told it necessarily.

"It's kind of like, going back to the flight analogy I just made. Wouldn't you want the captain to come on and say, 'We're going to have some rough turbulence but we should be done in about 20 minutes or so. So, if you just hang on and keep your seat belts buckled, it will be okay.' You know, to get some reassuring instruction with it, even though you can't change it. You can't open the door and get out of the plane, you can't exit, but there are definitely better ways to manage it and anticipate what is going to happen. That's half of the fear about knowing what you don't know."

Seeing one neurologist didn't provide what William felt he needed. "First, the neurologist really put a capstone on it and said, 'Well, you'll probably be like this for a while.' She came up with real generalities." He was concerned with the increasing number of lesions being spotted on repeated MRI scans.

"I'd ask, 'What does this mean?' She would say, 'They should level out at some point, and you'll probably be pretty fine.' I didn't know whether she had enough experience with people like me. The MS patients that I would see in her office seemed far beyond me; they were in wheelchairs and walkers and this was at a time before any of the ABC drugs (Avonex, Betaseron, and Copaxone) had come out. They had just started to come out. So, whoever had MS for a period of time before I walked in the door, got it pretty hard and pretty fast." He felt that they probably were treated with steroids and did not receive much medical treatment or complementary treatment that was very successful.

"Her experience was probably limited to that and she didn't have any experience with putting someone on an ABC drug to slow down the course of the disease. I was still in my mid-30s, and I walked in and I was still working at the time and she probably said, 'Well, he looks fine.' I think she felt like many people do. They think you look great. If you want to see me snarl and show my teeth, just say that.

"After all that I talked about and tried to share and I still heard people, especially those with MS, say, 'But you look great.' I'd think to myself, 'Thank you very much. I shave and I clean up real good.'"

William had a choice about his career options because he wasn't an employee, but there are individuals with MS who don't feel as comfortable about disclosing their illness. People with MS, of course, are in every occupational area, and not everyone is willing to allow their employer to know about a diagnosis of MS, even if it would be in their best interest to do so. Remember the young man in the MS group who hadn't dated in 10 years and now had to tell his employer about his MS?

One middle-aged woman struggled with her job in the entertainment industry. She believed that if she let anyone know, she'd be fired. Termination was definitely on her employer's to-do list, and she was almost fired because she began to forget important aspects of her job. In fact, she became so forgetful that staff complained that she left her car running in the garage beneath the building and was constantly losing things. But she looked perfectly fine to them, so they didn't have a clue what was happening to her cognition.

Much as her coworkers wanted to help, they couldn't keep covering up for her seemingly careless attitude, as they saw it, toward her duties. When the HR officer called her in for a discussion of her performance during the year and told her she was being given a remediation plan to improve her work, she realized that she couldn't hide her illness any longer.

For 2 years, she had lived in fear of being found out and preferred being referred to as "flighty" or irresponsible rather than let them know she had MS. She broke down and told them about her illness, and they began cooperating to change her job description and her duties.

She now works out of one location instead of several, has some support staff who double-check her work schedule for her and prompt her when she needs it. The condition no longer controls her and her work life.

What she hadn't realized was that she would have been covered, as she is currently, by the Americans with Disabilities Act (ADA), which entitles her to job accommodation. Much of her anxiety and depression about job loss, which she experienced on a daily basis, could have been averted if she had been knowledgeable about ADA and requested help.

Preferring to ignore the problem, she had never sought out information on her illness or her rights. In fact, she admitted to a fear of finding out what might be ahead for her in terms of her MS.

Stephanie, a College Student

ADA was the farthest thing from her mind when Stephanie, a straight-A student enrolled in accelerated courses while in high school, approached her freshman year at a major university. "I was really looking forward to going to college and now I'm not so keen on it. My experiences have been unexpected and my parents and I had to constantly remind the school of my legal rights."

Her rights included the school being required to give her extra time for tests, a quiet test-taking environment, making special arrangements for makeup exams when needed, and working to further her academic pursuits in whatever way her MS made it necessary. They didn't disregard her rights, but they appeared to be lacking in following the spirit of the law, and there was little understanding of MS students and their rights in the counseling offices.

"I had a flare-up and I had to take some time off and requested accommodation in taking a makeup exam for that." Her course professor refused to comply, and she had to remind college administrators that "I had the law on my side," she said. When they did schedule the makeup, "It was planned for the end of one of my classes that day, across the campus where I couldn't get there quickly and the extra time I was supposed to get was used in getting to that location."

It was all very stressful and anxiety provoking. When she brought this to the attention of college counselors, they indicated that the professor could do what he or she wished and that they had no control over it. There didn't seem to be an appreciation of advocacy on their part.

This was just one of many frustrating and depressing experiences during her first year at the school. She refused, however, to let it stop her. Now she is trying to maintain her motivation for school in the face of both depression and increasing anxiety. "I had been so excited and was so looking forward to going to college and now I don't." A course of psychotherapy was begun with a therapist with expertise in MS, and the possibility of medication to address both the anxiety and depression was under consideration.

Stephanie's MS started out, undiagnosed, as a series of recurrent bouts of severe nausea, tingling in her hands and feet, headache, and some other, seemingly unrelated problems. Her pediatrician didn't know what it was and at each visit to the office, a group practice, she was seen by a different physician.

"I had one attack and we didn't know what it was. It lasted about 2 weeks. I had uncontrollable vomiting and I was incredibly dizzy. My pediatrician thought I had a virus or something like that and I kept being treated as though I had a virus. There were even points at which we thought the virus was over but then, all of a sudden, I would start vomiting again. I hadn't eaten in probably a week and a half, and I couldn't walk.

"In the pediatrician's office, one person said I had migraine headaches. The reason I saw different pediatricians was that each person thought he or she had solved it as flu and then I saw someone else who thought it was migraine." The next trip to the medical office, she was seen by a third pediatrician.

It was this third physician who made the decision that hospitalization was the best course of action. "I didn't even know what was going on. I was happy that I was getting to go to the emergency room. I just wanted relief and I felt that this doctor was the first person who was really taking charge of the situation. He really knew what to do.

"They admitted me to the hospital and I was treated with antinausea medications. That helped so I was able to stop vomiting. The pediatrician said that there was a 99% chance that an MRI wouldn't show anything, but it did. Once they did the MRI and I got the diagnosis, I was treated with steroids."

When she got out of the hospital after a short stay, she went to a neurologist, who did a baseline study and found much of the lesion activity had cleared. The result was that she felt better and was doing well in school.

Her original physician then sent her to a pediatric MS specialist who decided the best treatment would be to be proactive with an initial treatment of interferon. She remains on this medication currently.

Some research indicates that cognitive deficits occur in over one-third of pediatric MS patients and academic accommodation is recommended to compensate for this impairment, which also affects verbal fluency. *Nearly half the children* in one study showed mood disorders. Attention and memory were the most frequent problems. The question remains, however, how frequent hospitalizations and a lack of sufficient research with pediatric patients affects current knowledge of MS in children in terms of depression and anxiety.

Children and adolescents with disorders like MS have not, as a group, been thoroughly studied and little is known about the course of their illness even though it's estimated that 2–5% of adult MS patients had the disease in their childhood. The incidence of both anxiety and depression, however, is noted, and children with chronic medical conditions may suffer from PTSD because of fears about their condition and their future. One factor that appears to stand out in the research with children is their anxiety regarding how MS will affect their social interactions, their schooling, or their career aspirations. Social involvement, however, was the primary concern.

One specialist in pediatric MS, Dr. Lauren Krupp, a neurologist and program director at the National Pediatric MS Center, Stony Brook University Hospital and Medical Center, has indicated, "I think that it's a problem that is underrecognized, although people are beginning to pick up on it now. In our experience, it's not something the kids are eager to come forward with, and it's more a matter of trying to draw it out of them."

How does it come to the attention of an MS professional? "Sometimes there are tears and we see kids who break down crying, sometimes there are issues with compliance in school or at home and sometimes there are problems primarily when the disease flares up."

The school nurse has been seen as especially helpful in many situations where the major problem may not have been noticed. "We've seen situations where the psychological problems were picked up by the school nurse, and it became clear when we had a psychologist see the child." At that point, the major issues were brought out and indicated a need for treatment.

Some children are teased by their classmates and become so depressed that swift action is called for. One child's classmates were teasing her that she had something wrong with her brain and, "As it turned out, the young girl did have a neurologic disorder; it's acute disseminated encephalomyelitis, usually a one-time problem, not MS, and the children had somehow heard about her illness."

In pediatric MS populations, Dr. Krupp indicated, there is an incidence of major depression of around 20%, which is higher than the general pediatric population. Often, Dr. Krupp indicated, there are compounding factors that may disguise the presence of MS such as adolescent adjustment issues that add an overlay of additional considerations into the mix. "So we're looking at school attendance, fatigue, moodiness, what kind of facial expression shows up on the neurological exam, and what kind of interaction takes place during the exam."

Generally, treatment is along the same lines as it is with adults and antidepressants are avoided, if possible, but sometimes are needed. When this occurs, a child psychiatrist is brought in to manage the treatment. "Counseling is something we try to provide for kids and their parents."

One major area that appears to be lacking in pediatric MS treatment is support groups, which Dr. Krupp feels would be extremely helpful. "We have a camp where kids with MS come together for about a week and they get tremendous benefit from being with other kids and trained counselors who know how to get the kids to participate in group activities. The kids who've had the disease for a while help the newly diagnosed. There are very few other camps around the country and ours was the first one." The problem with providing these outlets for kids with MS, Dr. Krupp explained, is that these are expensive activities and her hospital has to support them through fund-raising.

The question of exercise in kids with MS is problematic because "if they can do it, it's great but they may have to take a nap after school and that's when the sports activities are going on." The focus, as she indicated, is that "there are services for parents and kids and there is help through the National MS Society and our camp, and we do have a Web site (www.pediatricmscenter.org) that has information on support activities."

For Stephanie, MS still presents challenges. "I do get depressed and I do have a great deal of anxiety, currently." In addition to counseling sessions with a therapist, she is currently taking medication for both anxiety and depression. Prior to her diagnosis of MS, she had been treated for anxiety and she was taking medication for it.

If she were talking to another college student who had just been diagnosed with MS, she would recommend that they take the medicine because I know that a lot of kids are reluctant about taking medicines and also try not to be torn down by bureaucracy in school. That's something that's really hard to do.

"In school, people may not understand and you have to know that you may sometimes feel powerless and that's really frustrating. You have to realize that you're going to have to deal with professors who are not going to accommodate your needs."

Even though she had done all the appropriate things, there were still problems and hurdles that Stephanie had to tackle. "I did register for ADA and I knew what my rights were and I had a professor who refused to let me take a makeup test even though I had documentation for everything. All of the college advisors I went to told me it was fine; they took his side." This turn of events was a disappointment for Stephanie.

"I finally went to the dean of the college and she negotiated on my behalf. The deal was that I would have to take the test with less-than-24-hours' notice and they gave me a slot that I couldn't possibly make. They agreed I would come after class, but they made it at exactly the time that my class ended, in a location across campus, plus they put me in a noisy conference room. One of my accommodations was that I needed a quiet environment. I told the dean these things but she told me that I should just be glad that I got to take the test."

These experiences have been demanding and upsetting, but Stephanie has persevered. "I still haven't gotten over this experience because it was not fair." Her short college career thus far hasn't been without incident in terms of her MS, and Stephanie has had to be hospitalized while at school. It has happened more than once. "The first time I got sick at college, I had to go to the hospital. The second time, I needed accommodation; it was before the finals and the professor said I couldn't get extra time."

It was then that she realized that if she were going to get what was her right under the ADA provisions, she had to rely on her own skills, be proactive in her own behalf, and not depend on others. It was a quick lesson in resilience.

This was something she had never anticipated, but she refused to give in to the feeling of helplessness and powerlessness. "I had to call the dean and tell her that I had the law on my side. She said she was just concerned about my GPA (grade point average), so she told me to take the test and deal with it." These were not exactly comforting words for the young student with a diagnosis of a stress-exacerbated illness.

The dean had to appeal to the professor's supervisor and they finally gave Stephanie the accommodation the law requires. The professor told her it was a miscommunication. The situation didn't appear to be a miscommunication to Stephanie. "This was the person who the prior term had, again, refused to provide a makeup test for me even knowing that I had MS. It was the worst semester of my life. All the college counselor said about this matter was that I should go to therapy. The therapy office, when I called them, told me the problem wasn't me but the university and that there was nothing they could do about that."

Test taking and accommodation weren't the only problem at the college. "They wouldn't even give me my graded work back so that I could see what my grades were. I think my depression is coming from the fact that I haven't gotten over this mistreatment. I'm at the point now where I hate college. I had been so excited to go to college. I had a 4.0, I took accelerated classes, and studied all the time and now I can't even concentrate because I'm thinking about being in a university that doesn't care about me.

"The dean told me that they'd had, 'kids with MS and they've gotten through.' I told her I didn't want to 'get through,' I wanted to thrive.

"Medicine is for my depression and it's the depression that's really bogging me down. I think that might be leading to my inability to concentrate in class and my need to almost not concentrate and just take myself away. I think that in this case medicine might just get me back on my feet."

Despite all the challenges she's had to negotiate, she's proven that she could stand up for her rights, and she is working toward feeling better to do well in school and complete her degree. It hasn't been easy for Stephanie or her family to contend with the school situation and her illness at the same time, but the family has worked as an effective unit on her behalf.

Barbara, Wife and Mother

Barbara is an active young wife and mother who had never considered herself to be less than capable in any aspect of her many roles. "Seven years ago, I was having trouble with my hands and I kept thinking it was carpal tunnel. I had pain and tingling and it seemed like typical carpal tunnel issues. I remember asking the doctor, 'Could I possibly have MS?'

"For a couple of years prior to that, I remember being excessively tired. Something wasn't right but it was vague, and for a couple of years I would get well and feel okay. I was a woman and I had young kids and I was working and rationalizing everything. But I knew something wasn't right.

"One month later, I started having pains in my hip and they told me I had bursitis. Then within another month, my left leg went numb and I started getting pins and needles." The diagnoses kept coming. "So, they said the bursitis was pressing on a nerve in my hip. The only reason I can remember all of this is because I have my book out."

At the next symptom, yet another diagnosis was proposed. "About a week later, my right foot started going numb and by the time I got back to the orthopedist, I was numb up to my hip. They said I probably had a herniated disk.

"They did x-rays and, of course, that was fine and I had my first MRI and, of course, they were looking at discs. The orthopedist called a few days later and told me the discs were fine but that I had demyelination on my spinal cord." Having been a science major in school, she knew what that could mean. "So, I went to a neurologist and he confirmed it by another MRI of the brain and used contrast and tried to be reassuring that the orthopedist might not have been correct because it wasn't his specialty. He was reluctant but then he agreed that there was a lesion on my spine."

Barbara believes there's a need for greater education, especially about the cognitive problems associated with MS. "[I talked to] a lot of people . . . and I kept telling them that something was wrong. The original idea was that I had carpal tunnel and I asked if I could have MS and they kept telling me that since I didn't have any vision problems I didn't have MS."

However, the nagging feeling that there was something, something they weren't catching, kept haunting her. "I went through a course of steroids to get me through that and he did a spinal tap that came back normal. The neurologist indicated that something like 15% of the MS population had normal spinal taps. He indicated that since this was early in the disease, the spinal tap might not reflect it yet. He just followed me for a couple of years and within that time the left leg came out perfectly fine. Sometimes, I would have numbness or pins and needles and sometimes it would feel like bugs were crawling up my leg and it never fully healed. During that time I had other tests, including the optic nerve test and everything was normal."

She maintained her regular examination schedule. "Every 6 months, I went in for an MRI of the brain and then I switched neurologists. Three visits after the first flare-up, I had a couple of spots in my brain and they started getting a little bigger and there were a few small spots and they decided it was enough to say that it was MS. That was when I started therapy after I was officially diagnosed. Originally, I went on Copaxone and prior to that, they gave me Provigil for fatigue. After a time, I started having reactions to my medication and I was switched to Betaseron."

Her search for information on MS continued. "I went to a seminar, about a year after I started on the second medication. A friend of mine had been very stable on her medication for about 10 years and she didn't have a lot of residual damage and her neurologist was taking her off and monitoring her and seeing how she did. So, I started talking to my neurologist about that and we're actually trying that right now."

For the past 6 months, she has been off all medication, but she still takes Provigil for fatigue and multivitamins. "I know that the whole point of the medication is so that you're not having these silent attacks and building up damage. Since I'm being monitored, I know I can stop having those silent attacks and if anything happens, I can go back on my medications."

Fatigue came before any classic MS symptoms. "This is what was interesting. It was the fatigue and I didn't think it was a normal life fatigue because it was a whole body thing. It was cyclic, but it wasn't around the time of my menstrual cycle, but you could say, 'Well, it's your hormones.' It didn't follow that.

"It was that all of a sudden, every so often I would have this feeling that just walking was an effort and it would last a couple of weeks and I thought that maybe I had Epstein-Barr. Just walking was an effort. So, I thought I'd go to bed earlier, but it wasn't like I was just tired. It was totally different.

"My whole body felt heavy and worn out and I tried to exercise and work out, and usually after you work out you get back into a really good rhythm of working out and you start to feel better and I wouldn't. In fact, it actually fatigued me more and I'd come home and I'd be on the couch. That just wasn't right and then it would stop and I'd be back to my normal self and that's what bothered me."

The depression had come full force with her first MS flare-up. "The first attack was a very depressing time and that wasn't an underlying depression, it was a major depression. There were so many unknowns that I was numb. I couldn't drive; I was stuck in the house. I was depressed because I was very limited."

Mood fluctuations had been a part of her life prior to the diagnosis of MS, "and, of course, then there were the times of fatigue and that would just skyrocket with being blue, depressed and not feeling like I wanted to participate in normal activities that I enjoyed. After it was over, my mood improved, but when I was so fatigued, I felt limited and that would bring me down emotionally."

Barbara views herself as having a particular personality style. "I'm high strung and I had anxiety, very Type A and I put a lot of pressure on myself. If things didn't go right, I'd get upset. I was more frustrated than I was depressed.

"I had been put on an antidepressant during the first few years of my MS. When I go back for my next checkup, I'm going to talk about taking it again because I always feel there's something tugging at me. I thought it had passed and that's why I wanted to try to go off it, but now I'm reconsidering it."

Coping With the Cognitive Changes

Barbara has kept a journal of everything related not only to her MS, but all the other things that she needs to remember "because I have so many cognitive difficulties. I have to give my mother credit for that because she gave me a special baby book when my first child was born so that I could write down all the appointments I had for the baby. When I was diagnosed with MS, I decided to go back to that for myself and my appointments. It's been very helpful. Now I keep the records for the whole family and we make sure we get copies of all our medical records. That's one of my coping mechanisms. When I get frustrated because I can't remember something, now I know I can find it somewhere."

Her children have "been a huge help." She was first diagnosed when her youngest child was only a toddler and her other child was just beginning school. "I've been very fortunate that I haven't had a lot of physical issues and it's given my family some perspective and increased their awareness of things." She and her husband had to decide how to maintain "a fine line about how much we should tell the kids because we didn't want them to worry because it's such an unpredictable illness. Looking at it several years later, I'm better than I had anticipated that I would have been. I didn't want to pass my anxieties on to them.

"But my older child is very intuitive. He picks up things and catches on quickly. We did tell him what I had and tried to explain in terms that he would understand. We told him that it was affecting my nerves and how my body gets messages from my brain and we explained some of the things that could happen and he just went with it." They told him that his mother would have days where, "I'd be perfectly fine and there would be days I would need more help and days when I wouldn't be able to do anything." She thinks that it might have been different if she had had more physical problems, but her symptoms weren't readily apparent.

The family has further involved themselves and their children in events with the MS Society, and they have developed a deeper understanding of the disorder and its many manifestations. "As time has gone on, all of us have, as a result of the involvement with the MS community, relaxed a little bit and we aren't anticipating the worst. We know that if it does come, we know that we can deal with it. I know that tomorrow I could wake up blind, but it's not something that I think of every day. It's more what I have to remember and how to accomplish that."

Two Primary Aids

Two things that have been primary in Barbara's MS have been the cognitive problems and the fatigue. "Every Sunday night I sit down with the family wall calendar, my date book in my pocketbook, and I have to write out not only all the appointments or meetings, but also everything I have to remember to bring and what I have to do before any meetings. In other words, I have to put all the details down on a list and that has to go with me everywhere. Then I also have sublists. It works for me."

Lists aren't the only way she organizes and remembers things. "I have a voice recorder with me all the time. Sometimes, I'll just be driving the kids to baseball practice and you know you have to multi-task these days. In the past, I would think that I have to remember to get bread and milk. But now, 2 or 3 minutes later I know I thought about something and it may or may not be what I have to pick up at the store. I just know that I have to remember something and I have no clue what category it even falls into. I have no recollection other than knowing that I thought of something important.

"So with the voice recorder, if something pops into my head like that, I can just pull it out and record it and later on I can go back to it because I know there's something I have to remember. I keep it in a small pocket with my cell phone so I can get to it easily. I have to know I have that with me."

Everything has to be carefully planned in small steps in advance. "I always have to summarize things. Right now we're planning a dinner for one of the kids' groups and I'm in charge of planning this, so I have my to-do list for everybody.

"But for me, I have to break it down according to who's doing what. It doesn't matter whether that person knows he or she is doing that, *I have to know they're doing that particular thing*. Then I e-mail that person and tell him or her what I have down for him or her and I ask if I'm correct. So, I do constant checks and balances."

Socializing has been changed a bit since her diagnosis and the family doesn't do as much as they did in the past. "Even if we're having people over for dinner, which I used to do a lot more often, I have to sort it all out. Let's say I'm making three or four courses, I have to go over everything a day or two before and note how long each item will take to cook and that I'll have to start at a certain time and I have to do each prep step.

"I have to sit there and break everything down into small steps because I will either forget or get confused. That's been a big thing. If I try to look at the whole picture, I can't logically pull it all apart when I'm doing it. I have to think each piece through."

The sheer logistics of socializing has had an impact. "It's caused us to absolutely cut back on our socializing. I don't feel as confident in planning social events. My anxiety level goes up because I'm afraid I'm not planning it out right or I'm going to drop the ball. Even socializing at somebody else's house has gotten less comfortable because sometimes I can't think of words or people's names. It's more than, 'Oh, I'm not good with names.' It's there, but I just can't pull it out. It's the retrieval and it's frustrating because you know it's there, but it's slower. I'll get it, but I can't get it instantaneously when I need it and then I'm frustrated, so some situations I just avoid." She didn't express deep regret, but it was evident that it was something she missed.

Telling People About Her MS

"When I had the first attack, because I was numb and couldn't drive, I needed a lot of help with the kids and getting them to their activities. People knew something was going on and when they would ask how things were going and it was taking longer than we originally thought it should, my MS got out that way."

Her friends began to note the change. "There was also a mothers' group and I couldn't go to one of the meetings, and then when they all found out that it was possibly MS, the place was flooded with food and support. Ironically, I had just joined this club, and one of the other women had vision problems. Instantly, I knew what she had. She had been diagnosed sooner than me because, unfortunately, she's been more progressive. So, here in this group of about 30 women, two of us within a month were struggling with possibly having MS. Many people found out that way. They may have heard it through the kids' friends and people offered to help and it stunned all of us. That was early on with my core group of close friends."

The family has begun to become more involved in many MS-related activities. "For the last couple of years, we've done bike MS, so we send out letters to any contacts we have whether it's for baseball or scouts, so a lot of people who wouldn't have known have found out that way. It actually helped us as a family.

"I'm very open about the MS and it's actually been easier for me to be open about it since I don't have a lot of physical problems. When you look at me, you have no idea. So, when I'm tired or I slip up and it's not easy for me to communicate, it's easier for me if people know. Then they just know these things happen. If I'm in situations with people that I don't know that well, or I don't know them at all, or they may not know I have MS or how it manifests itself with me, I become anxious and those are the most difficult situations. I don't want people to think I don't care about something or to think poorly of me. Other people, they understand and they know when things happen and they just roll with the punches, as they say."

Barbara's immediate family and friends have been very supportive. "My husband is wonderful and whatever had to be done, we did it. That's just the way it is. My in-laws have been great. I have a huge support network with friends and neighbors helping me and my kids get places. Once I got through that initial attack and I was back to walking and driving, it was a lot easier. The kids were able to dress themselves, but one of my biggest frustrations was that I couldn't even go outside to throw the baseball around with them."

Planning activities that may be more physically taxing for her has been part of their family's approach to Barbara's MS. "There were things I couldn't do, but now I've learned to pace myself and if there's a fun activity that we want to do, I can work around that. We wanted to go to one of the big national parks and I wanted to be able to go there and hike and walk and at the end of the day, we'd come back and I'd crash and I was exhausted but it was good. We got through it. It was wonderful. They had a great time and, fortunately, they're able to do a lot of things for themselves. The older one is very self-reliant, he can help with anything that has to be done and he does it. He rises to the occasion and the younger one is getting there now so, fortunately, I don't have to run and do a lot."

Maintaining a Positive Attitude

How she has approached her MS has been one of Barbara's major tasks she set for herself. "Initially, I thought what a terrible curse for my children but we've been very lucky, we're blessed. We've gotten so many positives out of it that we wouldn't have had. The people at the MS Society are unbelievable with the things they've done to support us in terms of the family, and the whole MS community is incredible. Our community, our friends, our family have helped us see how lucky we are. We've met people who are in care facilities and they are brought to events by the MS Society where they participate. Without this organization they wouldn't have some of these opportunities because they don't have the family or social network of their own."

Maintaining active involvement in MS-related organizations and efforts on behalf of MS patients has proven to be a growth-promoting experience not only for Barbara, but for her children as well. "We've attended advocacy events in our state and one of my children came with me, and it was great because we got to meet legislators, we saw voting on the floor, and my son had a unique opportunity to see and meet people with MS. It really is a community that cares. We're all involved in finding ways to do positive things and to contribute to the whole MS community or health care in general and it's been wonderful. Our children have been able to be touched by all these other lives and it has proven to be a very positive influence on them. All of this helps offset some of the negative aspect of things.

"If I found out tomorrow or I go to the doctor next month and he said, 'Oh, we made a mistake. You don't have MS after all,' I would still keep doing the bike ride, still be involved, I would still be doing something for the MS Society. My son has a project for school that involves volunteering and he's thinking of doing something with disability awareness. These events have sparked awareness and an interest in doing something to raise the level of understanding about MS and other disabilities."

To raise awareness, even the Cub Scouts are using their jamborees to plan activities regarding disabilities. "They assigned disabilities to the scouts and they would maybe strap an arm to their side or put on blindfolds, or strap their leg and they had to use crutches. They even had things that mimicked cognitive deficits such as a tag flapping around in their face to distract them. Then they would have to do specific activities like those in wheelchairs had to try to get things off the top shelf, basketball, and it was unbelievable. I realized that's what we needed to do."

Speaking to her, you get the feeling that she has an excellent handle on her illness and how to best manage it within the context of her life. All the recommended steps are there from the family involvement to the social aspects of her life and how she maintains a positive attitude through it all. Despite the periods of depression that may come, Barbara still has a positive, upbeat attitude.

Spouse, Family, Friends, and Caregivers

Research has shown, repeatedly, that a strong family and social network help people living with MS and all of the firsthand stories you've read thus far confirmed this.

MS doesn't only affect the person diagnosed with it, as you've seen, but also has a residual effect on everyone who interacts with an MS patient. This vital social network, too, must be included either directly or indirectly in any life plan because all of them play a vital role in the outcome for treatment. Although they are not prescribed as part of a treatment plan, this active network provides a type of "medication" that can be central to maintaining the MS patient's quality of life and their mood. They are a major part of that resilience and sense of hope we mentioned earlier in this chapter.

Again, however, it has to be emphasized that caring for a loved one, in whatever role, takes its toll unless addressed adequately. Any life plan has to incorporate what research has indicated is the burden of a caregiver in any chronic disease.

In one study, caregivers indicated that the level of care, which they had to provide, had a negative impact on their interactions with friends, family, and even their careers. Consideration must be given, therefore, to attending to the needs of those who are in close relationships with an MS patient because they may contribute to the overall effectiveness of any treatment programs. Anyone with MS does not live in a vacuum and all programs require constant vigilance to this fact. If MS is a bidirectional communication disorder of the nervous system, there is also a bidirectional component in the social system.

How you react to your illness and how you decide to proceed are decisions that should be made after thoughtful consideration and discussion with those who care for you. The ride is going to be bumpy, no one can deny that, but these are bumps, not sheer cliffs. You will bounce back, you will continue with your life, and you can make decisions about your care.

Further Reading

American Psychological Association. *The Road to Resilience*. 2010. Available at: http://www.apa.org/helpcenter/road-resilience.aspx. Accessed February 2010.

MacAllister WS, Belman AL, Milazzo M, Weisbrot DM, et al. Cognitive functioning in children and adolescents with multiple sclerosis. *Neurol*, 2005;64(8):1422–1425.

Masten AS. Ordinary magic: resilience processes in development. *Am Psychol*, 2001; 56;227–238.

O'Brien MT. Multiple sclerosis: health-promoting behaviors of spousal caregivers. *J Neurosci Nurs*, 1993;25(2):105–112.

Ong AD, Bergeman CS, Bisconti TL, Wallace KA. Psychological resilience, positive emotions, and successful adaptation to stress in later life. *J Pers Soc Psychol*, 2006;91(4):730–749.

Sperry L. *Psychological Treatment of Chronic Illness: The Biopsychosocial Therapy Approach*. Washington, DC: American Psychological Association; 2006.

US Department of Justice. *Americans With Disabilities Act*. Available at: http://www.ada.gov/. Accessed December 28, 2009.

Weisbrot DM, Ettinger AB, Gadow KD, Belman AL, et al. Psychiatric comorbidity in pediatric patients with demyelinating disorders. *J Child Neurol*, 2010;25(2):192–202.

Wilks SE, Croom B. Perceived stress and resilience in Alzheimer's disease caregivers: testing moderation and mediation models of social support. *Aging Ment Health*, 2008;12(3):357–365.

Yi JP, Vitaliano PP, Smith RE, Yi JC, Weinger K. The role of resilience on psychological adjustment and physical health in patients with diabetes. *Br J Health Psychol*, 2008;13:311–325.

4

The "Ugly Twins" of Depression and Anxiety

Anxiety and depression never occur alone because, as we know, in almost every case we see both of them in anyone who indicates he or she is experiencing either depression or anxiety. They are what I call "the ugly twins."

Who could say that either of these emotions would be something that anyone would want to experience, whether occasionally or on an ongoing basis? Undoubtedly, they cause more problems than we can adequately assess with our clinical tools. Anxiety and depression bring each of us our own personal level of pain, whether physical or emotional, and no scale or clinical evaluation may effectively capture the degree to which we suffer. They are as personal as physical pain; they are totally subjective.

Both anxiety and depression are viewed as two of the most common emotions and psychological disorders in the U.S. population today. This may also be true for much of the industrial world, according to agencies evaluating world psychological disorders.

The ugly twins outpace most other medical illnesses in terms of the cost to business when we consider lost productivity and sick days allocated to them. To place this in a broader perspective, we can look at statistics coming out of the National Institute of Mental Health in the United States. Its calculations put the number of adults older than the age of 18 with a mood disorder in the millions, and the median age for mood disorders is 30 years old, which is close to the median age for the diagnosis of multiple sclerosis (MS). These statistics, however, are primarily for individuals who have received a diagnosis of depression or anxiety. The stats do not tell us about anyone who has a medical disorder and who is not receiving therapy or medications for a possibly associated depressive disorder. Therein lies the problem with statistics; they don't always "catch" everyone in their calculations. In addition, not all clinicians look for either of these diagnoses and they may go undocumented and untreated as a result.

Statistics alone are of little use when we are considering the reason behind a mood disorder, and so they fail to tell us much about what causes depression and anxiety. We do know that these are not simple, straightforward disorders. Many people will have a genetic predisposition to anxiety and depression, but they may never end up experiencing either.

One reason may be that these individuals have learned to cope in any number of ways; some of these are counterproductive to their health and welfare such as when they use drugs or alcohol. Some people may even deny that they have either disorder, preferring to suffer in silence, but nevertheless displaying symptoms to others. Environmental factors can play a role, too.

However, we also know that in the case of panic disorder, there appears to be a neurological component where a brain hormone is involved. The causes of depression and anxiety may be genetic or learned behaviors, and now we know that there are underlying medical conditions, such as MS and other autoimmune disorders, whose first symptoms may actually be depression and anxiety.

Stress can play an extremely important role in handling depression and anxiety for people with MS. Here, it is a question of not only learning to adapt to your changed physical and psychological circumstances, but also *learning new coping mechanisms* to help you help yourself and to modify your psychological outlook on life. These techniques may not have been part of any prior plan. Such an oversight can lead to a distorted negative belief about self-efficacy. If, as it is believed, it is vital to learn to contain or minimize stress in anyone's life, we know that it is of even greater importance for people living with a chronic condition because it may exacerbate symptoms of an autoimmune illness such as MS.

Some individuals with MS may suffer from mild depression for much of their lives and never seek any assistance with it, and therefore, they never receive a diagnosis of depression. Depression, however, does affect the quality of their lives and may, again, according to ongoing research, be an early indication of an inflammatory process even prior to a diagnosis of the presence of MS. There is now some evidence that is pointing to depression as a prediagnostic indicator of an underlying illness.

We know that fatigue is closely associated with depression and that in persons with MS, fatigue and depression were two of the most disabling symptoms noted from patients in a large study. Fatigue, in fact, had a major impact on the daily lives of individuals with MS who found that it prevented "sustained physical exertion, limits work and social role performance, and is related to lower quality of life." The reasons for the fatigue may be many, but it was felt that clinically significant depressive symptoms have a strong association with this impairment. The thought was, therefore: Treat the depression and lessen the fatigue.

There is, however, an additional physiological factor that must be taken into consideration and, now that we have the research to support it, we need to consider how the immune system plays a role in these autoimmune disorders. The mystery of how some of the disorders came to be is still one that perplexes scientists and this even extends to how depression and anxiety arise in these disorders.

In fact, in Alzheimer's disease, a disorder that some researchers feel may, in part, be involved with an inflammatory process, depression is one of the main components. For years, no one thought that depression in Alzheimer's disease should be treated and these patients were left to suffer from their depression almost in silence because they were losing their word-finding ability. They lacked the capacity to fully express what was happening to them and the depression also sapped their motivation to even try to verbalize their emotional pain.

Depression in patients with Alzheimer's often begins to manifest itself not necessarily as severe lack of motivation and lethargy initially, but as intense irritability, striking out, and unexpected rage reactions to inconsequential things in their lives. These were behaviors that were very alien to that person's usual personality. We now know that MS, too, has a component not only of inflammation, but also of possible damage to brain structures that help to mediate anger and reasoning ability.

One thing we do know also is that depression is a common feature of MS, so you are not alone. Anyone, not just persons with MS, who develops an autoimmune disorder may suffer from biologically driven depression. In fact, the National Institute of Neurological Disorders and Stroke indicates that it is both a neurologic and a neuropsychiatric disorder.

Over the past 20 years a great deal of research has been directed toward investigating depression and its biological basis, lifting depression from its former state of being a mental or psychological disorder. During the course of this research, it was discovered that there appeared to be a connection between depression and immunologically based disorders. The research evidence for this connection grows daily, just as there is now some evidence that a brain hormone may cause panic disorder.

Depression: The Biological Connection

When the immune system is activated by stress or by "invaders" such as bacteria and viruses or other substances that threaten your health, it initiates a ramped-up cycle of protection. The problem is that sometimes this protective cycle is disordered for unknown reasons. However, during the cycle, whether normally fighting invaders or abnormally damaging your body, certain chemical substances are produced by our protective white blood cells.

These substances (cytokines) are chemical messengers that produce changes in blood cells that combat infection. Think of them as police officers patrolling your body and looking for dangerous characters. They signal for reinforcements that immediately attack the invaders and then leave once control has been reestablished. In the normal functioning state of the immune system, there is a balance that is maintained by the various types of cytokines.

However, in autoimmune disorders, there seems to be a malfunction in the process. Instead of appropriately responding to invaders and then pulling back, the signal goes out for an increased and consistent attack, which results in inflammation. Normally, after the threat has been thwarted, the cytokines would calm down and return to their normal functioning of "watching the neighborhood." In the autoimmune disorder scenario, however, the defenders are on a rampage and seem uncontrollable. The reason for this disquieting and disordered autoimmune system is still not understood and the process that initiates it remains largely undiscovered.

A fuller discussion of the impact and the involvement of depression in MS was provided by Dr. Adam Kaplin, a psychiatrist at Johns Hopkins Hospital. Reviewing the evidence and the research on MS and depression, he found that "the available evidence suggests that depression in MS may result from immune-mediated effects on the brain." He goes on to say that there is no correlation "between the rate of severity of depression in MS and the degree of physical disability," which flies in the face of the idea that it is stress caused by increasing disability that is the primary reason for depression in people with MS. It is not because of a person's attitude that the person becomes depressed, but something else. Neither, he indicated, does genetics account for this depression.

Further, he pointed out that there is

> growing support for a role of cytokines . . . (in) depression, including . . . 1) various conditions that are associated with enhanced immune function . . . such as MS have a high incidence of co-morbid depression; . . . 2) the administration of cytokines to humans induces depression . . . ; 3) elevated circulating cytokines . . . are found in depressed patients; 4) elevated cortisol levels (the stress hormone) in depressed patients . . . ; 5) antidepressant drugs decrease cytokine and cortisol levels and can reverse the depressive symptoms induced by cytokine administration in . . . humans; 6) cytokines cause alterations in brain systems that have been implicated in depression . . .

The evidence, therefore, is consistent with out-of-control cytokines and an immune disorder in the rise of depression. It all suggests clinical management of depression as part of a treatment for MS where indicated. It is not a question of someone not having adequate coping strategies, nor of his or her having brought on the illness. The body, as one person stated it, "betrays" the person with MS. However, the outlook is not as dismal as this point of view may paint it. There are intense efforts aimed at finding the causes and devising more effective treatments for MS.

There are depression studies that point to changes in brain structure and size such as in the hippocampus, the section of the brain that controls learning and memory. Major depression alone can bring on problems in memory via these physical changes without the contribution of MS affecting cognition, but the autoimmune disorder component adds to it.

Depression and "Moral Failure"

Dr. Robert Sapolsky, a professor of biological sciences, Department of Neurology at Stanford University School of Medicine and a noted expert on depression, approaches the subject of depression and biology in a head-on fashion.

> Well, this is a huge problem of trying to get people to stop thinking of depression as a moral failing, a lack of will. When I'm lecturing, I always use a sound bite that goes, "Depression is as biological a disorder as is diabetes." I tell my students that you don't sit down a diabetic and say, "Oh come on, what's with this insulin, stop babying yourself, pull yourself together." In terms of the specifics of MS, an autoimmune disease, we have the hallmark of such a disease; hyperactivity of the immune system, including elevated secretion of inflammatory cytokines. That's great, perfect for the introductory immunology course. But there is a whole world of what these cytokines do in the brain that immunology people have zero knowledge of. They alter thermoregulation and appetite, they stimulate stress responses, and they disrupt learning and memory.
>
> There are explicit interactions between cytokines and the details of synaptic (nerve cell connections) plasticity. And on a similarly biological level, elevated cytokine levels increase the risk of depression. Have an overactive immune system and brain chemistry changes in a way that predisposes you toward depression; real biology here.
>
> The flip side, in terms of some standard treatments for MS, is, of course, glucocorticoids and they have their own biological link to depression. So the primary features of the disease can alter the biochemistry of depression, and the primary treatment can alter it as well.

As Dr. Sapolsky indicates, it's biology, pure and simple, not self-pity, not lack of will, not anything else.

Depression is seen as both a by-product of this change in the immune system of someone with MS, as well as a response to the changes that result and that the individual experiences. Therefore, it is both a biological action and a psychological reaction to the active disease processes.

This area of investigation, then, led to further work looking at which came first: the depression or the immune disorder. Some researchers believe it may be the depression that actually provides the first signal of an impending autoimmune disorder, but that has yet to be proven with solid research studies.

Handling the Depression and Diagnosis

Undoubtedly, you've experienced emotional changes, and you may have wondered if it was only you who felt that way. You may have been reluctant to ask others if they were experiencing these mood changes because there may have been an element of shame or insecurity about discussing it.

You may also have questioned whether you were weak, incapable of exercising the strength that you should have, or used some other means of looking at this mood change that was negative in its perspective. As William (see Chapter 3), who faced the diagnosis directly and questioned himself, told me

> . . . the frustration is that you look to yourself and wonder, "What did I do? What did I do to deserve this or what did I do to cause (it)?" I figured I had never done illegal drugs or anything like that. So I didn't think it was from some experience I had.
>
> I figured maybe I wasn't eating healthy, maybe I wasn't a good person, maybe I didn't pray enough. Okay, you start to wonder if this is God giving me a message or, what did I do wrong? The truth of it, and this is my truth, is that I didn't do anything wrong.
>
> This is the way that I was structured. If I had some preconceived problems within me, I didn't put them there. And if I did something to bring it out, whether it was a job or where I live or whatever, it was without intent. And, okay that's all interesting, but now you're stuck with it and you have to deal with it. Once I digested that it wasn't me or anything I had done, it became a waste of time to continue on that track. I did not deserve it and I don't think there's a single person with MS who deserved to have it. Nobody. Once I had that established, now what?

You may have felt the sense of guilt and inadequacy as this man felt. Let me reassure you that you have no reason to feel guilty because this is a biological process, as you can see by what he discovered himself. You haven't initiated it, as he also soon decided; your immune system did.

You may also have been told that this was "all in your head," as Anna (see Chapter 3) indicated a physician seemed to think, and that you had unresolved conflicts either earlier in your life or currently. As you remember she said she was in college and her symptoms came on suddenly. When she went for help, what she received was questioning about her current romantic life. The physician thought it might be related to a problem with her boyfriend. That's when she made that ringing statement about it "wasn't in my head, it was in my legs."

Although there may be cases where people with psychological problems do suddenly develop physical symptoms, that's not the case for anyone who has MS. People with MS live with a type of depression and anxiety that is directly related to autoimmune dysfunction. In other words, simply put, it's not "all in your head"; it's in your immune system, too. Of course, there can be some depression and anxiety associated with this diagnosis; there's no denying that, but it's not the be-all and end-all. Anyone who has ever received unexpected news that he or she had a chronic medical illness would have a psychological reaction to it. That's normal.

Sarah (see Chapter 3) didn't know if the depression she had been experiencing for years was related to undiagnosed MS or not. She began to reevaluate what had happened to her prior to her MS diagnosis and mentioned that she'd been treated, for years, for a depressive disorder. She'd taken medication for it and was still taking medication after her MS diagnosis. However, she never had any indication that there was anything physically wrong with her. Her belief, at the time was that it was something that would pass or that the physicians would prove themselves wrong when they did her spinal tap.

Her wish, however, didn't pan out and she did have to face her unexpected diagnosis. Sarah's world had changed in just a few days, but she was determined that she would not give up and that she would prepare, just like Barbara (see Chapter 3), for what might come.

A Missed Diagnosis

Some patients, like Anna, are led to believe that it's psychological and that they need psychotherapy to clear up the problem that appears to be hysteria. This idea was popularized in modern times by Freud who believed that there was a connection between a woman's psychological problems and her anatomy. We now know that this "wandering womb" theory was as wrong in Freud's time, as it was in ancient Greece where it was first conceived.

I knew a woman who was experiencing a variety of what appeared initially to be psychological problems. She was married and had three children, and after a consultation with a psychotherapist, it was felt that family therapy would be needed. The woman was losing her balance, complaining of vision problems, and had certain other difficulties with her memory and concentration.

When she was out in the bright sunlight, as well as when she took a hot shower, her symptoms would increase and she always had a feeling of depression and of being anxious because she was afraid of falling. The fear of falling was quite realistic because she had increasing problems with balance. The therapist found all of these symptoms as indications of a psychological dependence disorder and proceeded with that course of treatment for her and the family.

During the family psychotherapy sessions, which lasted for about 3 months, the woman was diagnosed as hysterical, seeking sympathy, somewhat self-involved, dependent, and less than mature. It was, for her, an extremely unpleasant and frustrating experience. No matter how hard she tried, she could not convince the psychotherapist that her symptoms were real and not psychological. Even an evaluation by the center's psychiatrist wasn't helpful. The therapy, ultimately, was terminated without a satisfactory result.

The family went off believing that the mother refused to change and was using these symptoms to manipulate the family members. The psychotherapist never thought a medical or neurological exam was indicated and did not refer the woman for one, even though her symptoms seemed to be making functioning increasingly difficult for her and she had to stop driving. Toward the end of the sessions, she was using her hand to guide her down the hallway in the mental health center. Again, this was seen as an act to engender more sympathy from the therapist and the family.

Three years later, the woman, together with her family, returned to the same community mental health center and the same psychotherapist, once again, for family therapy. The difference this time was that the woman had now been diagnosed with MS and all of her symptoms were truly physical and not psychological. The depression plus the symptoms, which would point to MS, were missed by several professionals involved in her care, including the psychotherapist and a psychiatrist to whom she was referred for an evaluation.

The woman's depression and her anxiety were very real and now the family had to come to therapy to learn how to deal with it. Their mother wasn't a woman who was self-centered and immature. Why did they return? Perhaps they returned to let the therapist know the true diagnosis and help her to deal better with those with medical illnesses like MS in the future.

For the mother, it had to be an affirmation that she had been telling the truth all along, but no one wanted to listen. The therapist, who normally didn't see patients with medical illnesses, had a preconceived idea of what was prompting the woman's symptoms and what she hoped to gain by them. The psychiatrist, too, appears to have been influenced by the therapist in his determination of her diagnosis.

This woman now needed to let the therapist and the psychiatrist know her accurate diagnosis. She also may have wanted validation because this unpleasant experience was connected to her self-esteem. Before, she had felt humiliated and helpless when she should have received support and understanding.

Depression resulting from MS doesn't have to be a one-way street. The good thing, if we can call it a good thing and I believe we can, is that the immune system is responsive to interventions that are both psychological and medical in nature. It's a two-way system of communication. A dysfunction of the immune system may set off the mood disorder and the anxiety, but that does not mean there is nothing that you, personally, can do about it. It's very possible that you can.

Learning to appropriately handle this depression, and to decrease the intensity of any depression you may be feeling, will have several positive effects on you, unquestionably. These effects may include decreases in pain severity, reduced stress, a possible decrease in the need for psychotropic medications, improved adherence to medical treatments, and increased motivation to make needed lifestyle changes such as diet, physical activity, and smoking cessation.

Depression Self-Test

Undoubtedly, you might be wondering whether or not you are depressed and, if you are, how depressed you might actually be. There is one way for you to get a nonclinical gauge of your level of depression.

In the 1970s, a researcher at the National Institute of Mental Health developed a self-assessment scale for depression called the CES-D or the Center for Epidemiologic Studies Depression Scale. This scale is a simple 20-item test, which only requires that you indicate how you felt on several variables *during the past week*. The ratings on the scale go from *rarely* or *none* to *most* or *all of the time*. We have included both the scale and the scoring so that you can take the test and score it yourself.

This depression self-test, as you can see, does not have items that deal with somatic or physical symptoms and is, therefore, a fairly good measure for anyone with MS. We've also provided a range of scores that may be used to get an estimated indication of the degree of depression.

Please note that no test should be viewed in isolation from the other factors in your life. No self-test can substitute for an appropriate and adequate clinical evaluation by a mental health professional. I would advise you that, if your score is in a range that indicates moderate-to-severe depression, you should consider having a consultation with a mental health professional to clarify your status.

This test should only be considered a *rough measure of depression* and might be used to help you to assess your progress as you begin to take steps to help yourself relative to any depression you may be experiencing. Again, it is *not* considered clinical it is only an aid in helping you to see what your mood may be currently and how it may change over time. It may even be helpful for you to begin to keep a chart of your scores as you begin to initiate changes in your life to help address your MS depression. In this way, it can be a motivator as well as an indication regarding where you may need to make some adjustments to some additional things in your life.

Circle the number of points next to the statement that best expresses *how you've felt over the past week.*

Center for Epidemiologic Studies Depression Scale (CES-D), NIMH

Points

1. I was bothered by things that usually don't bother me.
   a. Rarely or none of the time (less than 1 day)   0
   b. Some or a little of the time (1–2 days)   1
   c. Occasionally or a moderate amount of time (3–4 days)   2
   d. Most or all of the time (5–7 days)   3

2. I did not feel like eating; my appetite was poor.

    a. Rarely or none of the time (less than 1 day)   0

    b. Some or a little of the time (1–2 days)   1

    c. Occasionally or a moderate amount of time (3–4 days)   2

    d. Most or all of the time (5–7 days)   3

3. I felt that I could not shake off the blues even with help from my family or friends.

    a. Rarely or none of the time (less than 1 day)   0

    b. Some or a little of the time (1–2 days)   1

    c. Occasionally or a moderate amount of time (3–4 days)   2

    d. Most or all of the time (5–7 days)   3

4. I felt I was just as good as other people.

    a. Rarely or none of the time (less than 1 day)   3

    b. Some or a little of the time (1–2 days)   2

    c. Occasionally or a moderate amount of time (3–4 days)   1

    d. Most or all of the time (5–7 days)   0

5. I had trouble keeping my mind on what I was doing.

    a. Rarely or none of the time (less than 1 day)   0

    b. Some or a little of the time (1–2 days)   1

    c. Occasionally or a moderate amount of time (3–4 days)   2

    d. Most or all of the time (5–7 days)   3

6. I felt depressed.

    a. Rarely or none of the time (less than 1 day)   0

    b. Some or a little of the time (1–2 days)   1

    c. Occasionally or a moderate amount of time (3–4 days)   2

    d. Most or all of the time (5–7 days)   3

7. I felt that everything I did was an effort.

    a. Rarely or none of the time (less than 1 day)   0

    b. Some or a little of the time (1–2 days)   1

    c. Occasionally or a moderate amount of time (3–4 days)   2

    d. Most or all of the time (5–7 days)   3

8. I felt hopeful about the future.
   a. Rarely or none of the time (less than 1 day) 3
   b. Some or a little of the time (1–2 days) 2
   c. Occasionally or a moderate amount of time (3–4 days) 1
   d. Most or all of the time (5–7 days) 0

9. I thought my life had been a failure.
   a. Rarely or none of the time (less than 1 day) 0
   b. Some or a little of the time (1–2 days) 1
   c. Occasionally or a moderate amount of time (3–4 days) 2
   d. Most or all of the time (5–7 days) 3

10. I felt fearful.
    a. Rarely or none of the time (less than 1 day) 0
    b. Some or a little of the time (1–2 days) 1
    c. Occasionally or a moderate amount of time (3–4 days) 2
    d. Most or all of the time (5–7 days) 3

11. My sleep was restless.
    a. Rarely or none of the time (less than 1 day) 0
    b. Some or a little of the time (1–2 days) 1
    c. Occasionally or a moderate amount of time (3–4 days) 2
    d. Most or all of the time (5–7 days) 3

12. I was happy.
    a. Rarely or none of the time (less than 1 day) 3
    b. Some or a little of the time (1–2 days) 2
    c. Occasionally or a moderate amount of time (3–4 days) 1
    d. Most or all of the time (5–7 days) 0

13. I talked less than usual.
    a. Rarely or none of the time (less than 1 day) 0
    b. Some or a little of the time (1–2 days) 1
    c. Occasionally or a moderate amount of time (3–4 days) 2
    d. Most or all of the time (5–7 days) 3

14. I felt lonely.
    a. Rarely or none of the time (less than 1 day)   0
    b. Some or a little of the time (1–2 days)   1
    c. Occasionally or a moderate amount of time (3–4 days)   2
    d. Most or all of the time (5–7 days)   3

15. People were unfriendly.
    a. Rarely or none of the time (less than 1 day)   0
    b. Some or a little of the time (1–2 days)   1
    c. Occasionally or a moderate amount of time (3–4 days)   2
    d. Most or all of the time (5–7 days)   3

16. I enjoyed life.
    a. Rarely or none of the time (less than 1 day)   3
    b. Some or a little of the time (1–2 days)   2
    c. Occasionally or a moderate amount of time (3–4 days)   1
    d. Most or all of the time (5–7 days)   0

17. I had crying spells.
    a. Rarely or none of the time (less than 1 day)   0
    b. Some or a little of the time (1–2 days)   1
    c. Occasionally or a moderate amount of time (3–4 days)   2
    d. Most or all of the time (5–7 days)   3

18. I felt sad.
    a. Rarely or none of the time (less than 1 day)   0
    b. Some or a little of the time (1–2 days)   1
    c. Occasionally or a moderate amount of time (3–4 days)   2
    d. Most or all of the time (5–7 days)   3

19. I felt that people dislike me.
    a. Rarely or none of the time (less than 1 day)   0
    b. Some or a little of the time (1–2 days)   1
    c. Occasionally or a moderate amount of time (3–4 days)   2
    d. Most or all of the time (5–7 days)   3

20. I could not get "going."

    a. Rarely or none of the time (less than 1 day)   0

    b. Some or a little of the time (1–2 days)   1

    c. Occasionally or a moderate amount of time (3–4 days)   2

    d. Most or all of the time (5–7 days)   3

TOTAL POINTS =

SCORING: Circle the score next to your response for each question, add up all the points you've indicated for the questions. Possible range of scores is 0–60 with higher scores indicating possible presence of more symptomology.
(Source: National Institute of Mental Health)

The scoring for this test is as follows:

CES-D Scoring

0–15 suggests *minimal or mild depression*

16–21 would indicate *mild to moderate depression*

Above 21 suggests the possibility of *major depression*

As you look at your score, please remember what I noted previously; these scores are *not* to be interpreted as though they were derived from a thorough professional, psychological evaluation. They can only provide *rough estimates* and should be discussed with a mental health professional if there's an indication of depression. If you do decide to use the scale, you may want to keep your treating physician or neurologist advised and you can even provide scores for them, if so desired. This way, both of you can look at your status.

Stress and Depression

Stress, in the case of anyone with MS, has been found to be a critical factor in relapse to some degree. Research has shown that stressors may be involved not only in relapses, but also in the number and severity of relapses. The connection, however, has not been found across a sufficient number of studies to make this a hard-and-fast rule of the relationship between stress and MS relapse. What can be said is that, as it is with any illness, stress is something that patients need to minimize and work on in a constructive manner to optimize their health.

Discussing stress requires, I believe, consideration of something else: smoking. One word on smoking might be helpful here because stress and smoking appear to also have a strong relationship.

One of the reasons people smoke is not only that nicotine is addictive, but also it is a mild anxiolytic substance, meaning it can "treat" mild anxiety and help someone calm down. Now you can understand why, in social situations, there is a greater tendency for people to want to smoke. So if you're a smoker, and you have had a great deal of difficulty stopping, you now know another reason for a roadblock in your way: social anxiety. I've heard it said that smoking addiction is just as bad as heroin addiction in that it is extremely difficult to "kick."

One recent study of people with MS who were smokers indicated that smokers appear to have 17% more brain lesions, 13% larger ventricles (large open spaces in the brain that serve specific functions), and a smaller brain size when compared to nonsmoking individuals with MS. The lead researcher on the investigation, Robert Zivadinov, writing in the professional journal *Neurology*, expressed the belief that this study demonstrated "that smoking can promote brain tissue injury in multiple sclerosis patients," and he indicated that this was a significant finding.

These researchers believe that smoking is "an important contributor to disability progression in patients with MS." There was some suggestion that smoking may cause greater risk for disruption of the blood-brain barrier, our body's natural protection against disease-promoting substances. This usually robust blood-brain barrier, in theory, provides the biological highway for the entrance of MS-promoting materials even without smoking, so smoking would further enhance the ability of these substances to enter and cause even more damage to the brain and the central nervous system.

Another study, also published in the journal *Neurology*, found that smokers had significantly more severe disease and that their disease progressed at a faster rate. Experts in the field of neurology viewed this research as providing a compelling reason for people with MS to stop smoking as a means to provide additional self-treatment for their disease.

Some people with MS who are smokers, in an effort to alleviate their anxiety and pain without prescription medications, have begun turning to smoking marijuana. We know that this drug has anxiolytic properties and may alleviate pain, but it carries with it a host of unknown dangers; two, of course, being lung and stomach cancer. One of the other dangers of this drug is that it can lead to serious psychiatric problems.

The therapeutic prospects of marijuana as a useful aid for patients with MS have been recognized by the National Multiple Sclerosis Society in one of its *Expert Opinion Papers* articles entitled, "Recommendations Regarding the Use of Cannabis in Multiple Sclerosis." The Society, however, indicates that although an estimated 15% of people with MS are using marijuana for symptom relief, the organization is not recommending its use because of both legal barriers and insufficient studies that would clearly demonstrate benefits comparable to existing therapies.

Although there may be insufficient studies to demonstrate benefit for patients with MS, more than a dozen states, as of this writing, have legalized the use of medical marijuana for people with certain chronic diseases, including MS. New Jersey, in 2009, was the most recent state to change the law regarding marijuana use for medical purposes.

Fighting Depression

Decreasing depression can bring about an enriched sense of social interactions and relationships and, of course, those all-important changes in the immune system. Depression may be at the root of several problems in your life, and it is one area that requires focus and work on your part. Nevertheless, it's well worth the effort. How many times have you worked hard to help others achieve their goals or to have a more comfortable life? Now it's your turn, but this time you're going to be working toward your own goal.

We know that socialization can be an important factor in depression and anything that can be done to make socialization possible or more enjoyable is all to your benefit. One of the primary symptoms of depression is that it causes people to isolate themselves and to eliminate or severely cut back on social interactions. This self-imposed isolation continues to build and with it comes an increased sense of anxiety related to going into social situations and a feeling of both ineptness and inertia. Together, the ugly twins of depression and anxiety work intensely against your best interests.

One gentleman told me that, "I'm not sure that I have depression because when I think of depression I think of a depressed state; woe is me, things aren't going to get any better, I might as well be dead. That is not me. There are certainly the ups and downs in my life. Some days are better than others, something I struggle with daily, routinely. . . ."

However, he also indicated that he was going out less and less and that his wife has to think of things that need to be done, such as going to the post office, and she made it his "assignment" to do them—just to help him get out of the house more. He continues to struggle and he knows that "MS and what a person must live with can be very depressing if we don't help ourselves to improve ourselves." He's actively working toward that goal.

He had also indicated to me that when he finally received his diagnosis of MS, he began to have marked shifts in irritability and angry outbursts. At the time, he didn't view this as a form of depression, which it well may have been or, as some researchers hypothesize, it could be indicative of some brain involvement caused by MS.

Look at what else depression does to you and what its symptoms are. The symptoms include feelings of a lack of worth, decreased energy, decreased motivation, a decrease in your self-esteem, feelings of sadness, guilt, loss of interest in pleasurable activities, problems in concentration and memory, changes in both sleep and appetite, feelings of both hopelessness and helplessness, and even physical pain in some people. That's a long list and it's only one "face" of depression because it has two faces: one sad, the other mad.

Consider what one or two of those symptoms can do to you in terms of your ability to function in your daily activities plus the fact that MS is sapping your energy. Then, when you consider how it affects your self-esteem, you'll see that depression is one of the major roadblocks to your continuing through on your medical care. Left unchecked, depression may only worsen and further incapacitate you. There are going to be days when depression will whisper in your ear that, "You can't do that," or "You shouldn't do that," or "You don't feel like it, do you?" Don't listen to either of the ugly twins. Take time out to break the cycle.

It's important to fight depression at every opportunity. Depression is truly one of the more serious of the psychological problems you will face in your life. And again, remember that you're not alone because we know that depression affects literally millions of people worldwide.

In fact, the National Institute of Mental Health in the United States estimated in 2004 that about 57 million Americans older than the age of 18 suffered from one specific mood disorder—depression.

The actual number of people experiencing depression may be much greater. There is still a stigma surrounding depression and other psychiatric disorders. Many people with whom I've interacted on a professional level mentioned that they are ashamed to indicate they are depressed because they see it as a weakness or they're afraid they'll be put into a psychiatric hospital. Believe me, it's not 1920 and it's not easy to get anyone into a psychiatric hospital these days unless they are truly a danger to themselves or others.

It's not a weakness, it is a serious disorder, and it is widespread. The U.S. government's estimates are that by the year 2020, depression will be both a serious and prevalent illness, second only to heart disease. That's a pretty shocking prospect.

If you suffer from depression, and most people with MS do as you've already seen, let me tell you that you are fighting very real anxiety and depression caused by very real changes in the body. As you've seen and read what others have said, they are not changes brought on because of any deficits in personality or an inability to fight this mood change. There's no question that it's a struggle.

Depression is part of a triad that is composed of depression, anxiety, and pain. Therefore, when you fight depression, you are also fighting for freedom from as much pain as possible and from the grip of anxiety. Anxiety, on its own, intensifies pain, so decreasing anxiety and stress and promoting relaxation helps with pain. We know that for many people living with MS, pain is ever-present and narcotic medications may not be acceptable or effective enough for everyone. All three members of this triad have a highly negative effect on your self-esteem, your ability to handle stress, your immune system, and your daily functioning as well.

Depression is also a disorder that may require multiple techniques to address its many symptoms. So, please, be good to yourself and remember the quotation from an ancient philosopher that begins, "If I am not for myself, then who will be for me?" This is not selfishness; this is good common sense. There will be days when you won't feel like being good to yourself or others, so just keep this proverb in mind and, maybe, write it down and keep it with you.

Caring for yourself is one of the most important things you will do. If you care for yourself, then you can care for others and you can be involved in their lives and your own life in a fuller fashion.

The Psychological Component

If you experience depression, whether it's initiated by changes in your body's biology or your reaction to these changes, there are several things to be considered.

Depression is like a veil that is thrown over your mind and that affects both your mood and your perception of things in your life and of yourself. The change may appear to come almost unexpectedly with no rhyme or reason, leaving you wondering what is happening. However, one of the things that will happen is that you will become less joyful and all of your activities will be colored by depression. There's a good reason that it's referred to as a "blue mood."

Even enjoyable activities will begin to take on a negative cast and deprive you of the enjoyment inherent in them. If this depression persists, it will widen into causing you to become irritable, short-tempered, even affect your concentration and memory.

Once concentration and memory are affected, your attention span will suffer. You may begin to question yourself because of these changes in concentration and memory, but there's one very important thing to remember. The important thing here is that attention and concentration go hand in hand and if you can't concentrate, you will have difficulty forming memories. The three basic components of memory all work together: attention span, concentration, and memory. For this reason, it's the "gold standard" used by the Social Security Disability evaluators when they look at someone's ability to work. They call it PPC (pace, persistence, and concentration).

Undoubtedly, there is a biological factor in memory or cognitive functioning in MS because of the injurious plaques that we know form in the brain, so we can't ignore this fact. The brain, however, has many pathways to enable memory and even people with severe strokes, given sufficient time and therapy, can regain more function than had previously been thought. There are literally billions of cells just waiting to be put into service or back into service, if they've been put "off line" by some physical impairment in that master organ.

The result of deficits in these three factors (attention span, concentration, and memory) can, again, attack your sense of self-esteem, capability, and confidence. You may begin to believe that you are losing your memory and this can be a self-fulfilling prophecy. You expect yourself to not have a good memory, and then it happens. This reinforces your belief that you have memory problems and this belief will make it appear that any memory difficulty is worse than it really may be. Can you see the cycle here? It's like the proverbial tail wagging the dog.

When you begin to say things like, "Oh, I can't remember, exactly," or "That's too much for me to remember," your brain "hears" this and retains this negative statement about you. Each time you come across an instance when it requires that you remember something, you can easily fall into the trap of thinking that you can't do it. Step back. Give yourself a break here. No one can remember everything *instantly*. What's wrong with learning new memory tricks?

Now the other ugly twin begins to march out on your life's stage and play its role. When you think you have memory problems, you also develop anxiety around this perceived difficulty or lack of ability. Anxiety disrupts your ability to concentrate because it attacks your belief system about yourself, so you have more problems remembering than you would if you didn't become anxious.

Don't put yourself down. Too many people in this world are just waiting for a chance to do it for you. Whenever you begin to feel that way, understand that there will be times that your memory may not be as sharp. However, that does not mean that you are going to lose your memory entirely. Stay tuned because in the next chapter and in Chapter 7, you're going to learn ways to handle memory, anxiety, and even improve social interactions.

None of us remains as sharp as we may have been in the past and this is for various reasons. One reason is that as adults, we begin to have many more demands made of us and much more information must be quickly consolidated and retained. Information that doesn't seem as important or even significant for us to retain can quickly slip out of our short-term memory and not be placed into those long-term vaults we have in our brain. Memories that were once clear, however, aren't lost. The connections to them may have weakened and they just need a bit of retooling to get them back in form. You can relearn information you once used in the past faster than you can learn something entirely new. This proves that it's still there. Forgetting may be more of a matter of displacement than disappearance.

One interesting fact about memory, which I might mention here, is that one of the best times to work on memory is during sleep. Yes, while you're asleep. We know that studying or reading important material *before you go to sleep* is a very good method to assist in retaining information and placing it into long-term memory. Getting a good night's sleep, as you can see, is also an important aid to memory and a way of fighting anxiety and depression. Inadequate sleep fosters anxiety, depression, and increasing irritability, too.

During the day, distraction plays a great part in memory, and depression keeps you distracted. You don't want to focus on much because you don't have the motivation to do so. So, you don't attend, you don't concentrate, and you don't take in what you might have before. Depression can also affect memory by affecting your energy level, which has a direct effect on your motivation to do things. How motivated, do you suppose, a tired and depressed person could be? What would be the result? Doesn't MS also sap your energy level? So, if you want to do something of a mental nature, what might be the optimal time for you to pick to do it? Choosing the late afternoon or evening rather than the morning might be setting yourself up for failure.

You may also find yourself frequently depressed for no reason and wonder whether life is really worth all this suffering. If this goes on for weeks or months, it is an indication that professional help should be considered. Again, this is not a sign of weakness, but rather a sign of strength and motivation to fight depression. There is no reason not to share your feelings of depression with others, whether they are family, friends, or mental health or medical professionals. People want to help you, so reach out and allow them to be there for you in your time of struggle. Yes, it may take a little getting used to, especially if you're someone who has always prided yourself on your independence and your ability to do everything for yourself.

I'm sure that you have had moments of doubt about yourself, but that does not mean you suffer from depression. Doubt is normal and we all have doubts at one time or another. Depression is more of an overreaching sense of sadness, and it generally does not come and go quickly. Being sad about something or responding to something that is hurtful and becoming somewhat sad as a result is normal. It's more of a reaction of what you're feeling at that point and you may feel depressed, but there's a reason for it. Look for the positive not the pathological.

In fact, "normal" itself means a full range of moods and emotions, and depression is one of those normal moods. It's not abnormal to feel depressed once in a while. If you were never depressed, we might begin to wonder if there was another problem.

Life in this respect can be compared to a complicated food dish that we create where depression would be one of the spices we add to this dish. This "spice" alone might be bitter, but when placed in the completed dish, it complements the other ingredients and provides a balance of flavors. The total elimination of depression would be abnormal because it would mean we don't respond emotionally to anything. In fact, it's the reason some people don't want to take any type of antidepressant medication—because they think it will make them incapable of emotion. Not so. Others think, "I'll get addicted." Not so. Antidepressant medications are not addictive. Yes, your body can acclimate to any medication and weaning yourself off of it can produce some withdrawal symptoms, but that's to be expected. Your body has learned to function with this medication and now you're telling it that it's not going to have it anymore. Adjustment is now in order and your body has to adjust.

I believe that depression can point out for us the joy in life as it allows us to see the other side. Therefore, it does have its place in putting things into perspective and can even be a motivator to return to that more pleasant existence we all seek. As a psychologist, I know that anxiety, too, has its place in a normally functioning life. Anxiety, in appropriate levels, pushes us to create, learn, and work toward goals. Any motivational psychologist can tell you that.

It is when anxiety is out of all proportion to what we are experiencing that it has its most devastating effect. The one thing that we always attempt to do is maintain an appropriate level and to quickly cut off anxiety when it begins to escalate. Just as pain must be managed quickly and efficiently when it first begins, anxiety, too, must be managed in the same way. Anxiety and pain are very similar. Both anxiety and pain, if left unmanaged, can become unmanageable. The best intervention is quick and conservative.

As we've also seen in the research, pain and anxiety appear to have some of the same underlying biological aspects, and managing one can lead to managing the other. It's a relationship where bringing down anxiety can result in bringing down pain. In addition, we know there's often pain associated with MS and, therefore, containing anxiety can be beneficial in terms of pain relief.

When there is a diagnosis of a chronic medical illness, undoubtedly we feel somewhat depressed and anxious, and that's normal. We may even feel this mood change for several days or even a few weeks as the realization comes that there are things that we can do and there are treatments available to us. However, it takes a bit of time for that understanding to come to us. Initially, it can be overwhelming and that, too, is common.

If I had a word of advice here, I'd tell you to do as I've always told my students. Don't make any important decisions the first thing in the morning; don't make them on Mondays and let everything, if you can, have a bit of time before you act. This doesn't mean you're a procrastinator. It means you're permitting yourself to adjust, seek answers, and make informed decisions, not be impulsive as you may find you're apt to do.

Anxiety's Role

Once anxiety strikes hard, there's a secondary wave that may be waiting to punch you. That's when anxiety brings out the big guns of panic attack. The result of this type of attack can result in your being afraid you'll have another attack. You will begin to avoid doing things or being in places where you had the first attack. It may even stop you from going to much-needed physical therapy or continuing with treatment at some point. The main problem here with anxiety, with its panic component, is that it can begin to foster phobias. One such phobia can be related to injectable medications. Needle phobia is something we see in patients who must give themselves medication via this route.

Any experience that results in some unpleasantness, say learning to inject yourself, or isn't as easy as you thought it might be may provide the fertile environment for phobia. You may have had fears that you weren't prepared to face or something happened that was unexpected. Panic tries to take your legs out from under you and leave you defenseless. It's nasty, it's stealthy, and you may not recognize it because it can disguise itself as something akin to a heart or lung problem with labored breathing, racing pulse, and profuse sweating. In fact, it's often mistaken by people having one of these attacks as a heart attack.

If left untreated, panic/anxiety can result in your not using your medications appropriately or becoming housebound and socially isolated. No one wants that and certainly, it's not something that you would choose for yourself. We know that socializing is like a medicine for the soul, so be sure to make it a part of your everyday life as much as you can.

The ugly twins are now on your radar, so keep watching for their appearance. In the following chapters, we are going to provide several ways that will enable you to effectively exercise some control over the ugly twins. You don't have to come up with things on your own because we are going to be there to support you with examples of what others with MS have done to wage this particular battle.

Keep in mind that your resolve may fluctuate as the results may fluctuate, too. No journey in life is in a straight line. There are going to be some ups and downs, and the best way to handle them is to prepare yourself in advance and to keep that in mind. There will be some setbacks and there will also be successes.

Concentrate on those successes, no matter how small they may seem to you. Each success is to be applauded, not belittled. Give yourself credit and know that even a very small success is worth your being proud of it. When you do this, you are fighting the ugly twins.

Yes, you will be a little anxious, and you may even wonder if you can do it. You may question how these methods could possibly work. That's the ugly twins working against you, again. Just toss caution to the wind and do your best. *There's no losing here, only winning, and you're the one who gains.* The thing to do is to try and try your best. Don't give up. You're important. You're worthwhile.

Need a laugh here? Just remember *The Little Engine That Could* and what that little engine kept saying. Remember, "I think I can, I think I can"? Put another way, it's positive anticipation and perhaps even a self-fulfilling prophesy.

You may not be able to do everything and that's okay, too. Do as much as you can, and then, if you want, try the things that weren't so successful again. Sometimes the second time around can be the charm. Did you ever know anything worthwhile that didn't take practice? Whatever you've learned in your life, beginning with the alphabet and reading those little primers all the way up through any skills you may have perfected, required practice, and this does, too.

You're going to be the judge in evaluating what your best effort is and you're going to be the one to give yourself a pat on the back when you know you deserve it. Let the anxiety associated with trying, as I said before, be a motivator, not an impediment.

I knew a man who, because he was embarrassed, had never learned to swim as a youngster, never went on family trips to the beach or lake, and never went to parties or outings with other students. He always made excuses about having to work. He had graduated at the top of his class from college, was on the boards of directors of major corporations, and was successful in business, but he had that basic fear that someone would find out he couldn't swim, he was afraid to take a plane, and he couldn't play any sports. He'd spent his entire childhood studying to maintain his grades and used that as a reason for not joining friends in sports. Actually, his life was ruled by an anxiety disorder, but he never admitted it to anyone.

One day, when he saw his young son jump into a pool and giggle as he bobbed up, he decided to face his anxiety. He hired a swim coach who gave him private lessons and he took off. Not only did he face that fear, but he also tackled skiing, ice skating, tennis, and everything he could fit into his schedule. Next, he accepted a promotion that required frequent plane travel. No, he didn't have any physical illnesses, but he had been hobbled by severe anxiety and the fear of "looking foolish," as he phrased it, even though he had a high-level executive position at an international corporation. Later, even complicated major cardiac surgery couldn't stop him. He'd faced his demon. Looking back, he realized how his fear of looking foolish had led to his missing out on many wonderful social opportunities and he was determined not to let that happen again. The last time I heard about him he was jumping out of helicopters to ski down mountain slopes.

The fear of appearing foolish keeps many people from engaging themselves in opportunities for making significant changes in their lives; that also applies to not entering rehab programs for MS or therapy groups. Each day is a special opportunity that needs to be used because, once it's gone, you can't recapture it and no one wants to worry about "what might have been."

Remember, the Robert Burns' poem indicates "the best laid plans of mice and men often go astray." They may go astray but that doesn't mean we lose our ability to *reconstruct a new plan* that fits into this new set of circumstances. Burns was telling us to be prepared for what may come because change is always in the wind. John Greenleaf Whittier reminded us, "For all sad words of tongue and pen, The saddest are these, 'It might have been.'"

Further Reading

Answers.com. Medical encyclopedia: hysteria. Available at: http://www.answers.com/topic/hysteria. Accessed April 2010.

Bremner JD, Narayan M, Anderson ER, Staib LH, Miller HL, Charney DS. Hippocampal volume reduction in major depression. *Am J Psychiatry.* January 2000;157(1):115–118.

Chwastiak LA, Gibbons LE, Ehde DM, et al.Fatigue and psychiatric illness in a large community sample of persons with multiple sclerosis. *J Psychosom Res.* November 2005;59(5):291–298.

Dantzer R, O'Connor JC, Freund GG, Johnson RW, Kelley KW. From inflammation to sickness and depression: when the immune system subjugates the brain. *Nat Rev Neurosci.* January 2008;9(1):46–56.

Gandey A. Smoking linked to lesions and brain shrinkage in multiple sclerosis [Medscape Medical News Web site]. August 20, 2009. Available at: http://www.medscape.com/viewarticle/707749. Accessed December 23, 2009.

Gold SM, Irwin MR. Depression and immunity: inflammation and depressive symptoms in multiple sclerosis. *Neurol Clin.* 2006;24(3):507–519.

Kaplin A. Depression in multiple sclerosis. In: Cohen JA, Rudick RA, eds. *Multiple Sclerosis Therapeutics.* 3rd ed. London: Informa Healthcare; 2007:823–844.

National Institute of Mental Health. Runaway vigilance hormone linked to panic attacks *Science Update.* December 28, 2009. Available at: http://www.nimh.nih.gov/science-news/2009/runaway-vigilance-hormone-linked-to-panic-attacks.shtml. Accessed September 15, 2010.

National Multiple Sclerosis Society. Recommendations regarding the use of cannabis in multiple sclerosis. *Expert Opinion Paper.* Available at: http:// www.nationalmssociety.org/PRC. Accessed December 2009.

Pucak ML, Carroll KA, Kerr DA, Kaplin AI. Neuropsychiatric manifestations of depression in multiple sclerosis: neuroinflammatory, neuroendocrine, and neurotropic mechanisms in the pathogenesis of immune-mediated depression. *Dialogues Clin Neurosci.* 2007;9(2):125–139.

Radloff LS. The CES-D scale: a self-report depression scale for research in the general population. *Appl Psychol Meas.* 1977;1:385–401.

Raison, CL, Capuron L, Miller AH. Cytokines sing the blues: inflammation and the pathogenesis of depression. *Trends Immunol.* January 2006;27(1):24–31.

5

Learning to Help Yourself

There are many ways to approach the matter of self-help. In fact, there are several terms currently in use for this form of, if you wish to use the term, self-therapy. Some people refer to it as bodywork, others refer to it as mindfulness, and still others just call it self-help or self-improvement. I'm not sure I agree with the term *self-improvement* but I am willing to accept it as a useful term in the context of improving the quality of your life. We know that quality of life is extremely important and that one of the things that disorders such as multiple sclerosis (MS) hits hardest is someone's sense of his or her quality of life. When this happens, the result can be a feeling of extreme loss, anger, fear, or a sense of one's helplessness in the face of a chronic and serious illness. But that doesn't have to be the case.

The thing to do, and the challenge here, is to look for ways where you can make a difference and then create a simple plan of action that will work for you. Start off slowly and see how it goes. If you progress and feel you've accomplished something, consider adding something else. Always keep in mind that no one is grading you; you are the one who decides what you can do and how far you're going to reach. But do keep in mind that trying to carve out overachieving goals may not be in your best interests. Small, simple, and easy does it are much better in the long run.

There are things that you can do that have been shown to be effective not only in lowering levels of anxiety and depression, but also in raising your awareness of the abilities that you do have. Once you begin to use these techniques and benefit from them—perhaps just a bit at the beginning—you will begin to experience a change in your beliefs. You will see that you are more capable than you thought, and it will begin to lift that burden of depression and that feeling of insecurity that may have overwhelmed you. In psychology, we have a saying that is, "First the behavior, then the belief." In other words, once you find that you are capable of a certain behavior, your belief system about your ability and that behavior will change. Optimism can replace pessimism.

Some of the things that we will discuss in this section may seem new to you, others will be ones that you may have heard of, and still others may be things that don't really seem, on the surface, like effective self-help techniques. But they all are. Everything that we will present in this chapter is based on research studies and the clinical experiences of specialists in the field of psychological rehab in terms of anxiety, depression, and pain relief.

When I say "pain relief," you may be wondering why it's been mentioned in this section. People who have MS experience pain, and some have felt that there was little outside of medication that they could take to relieve this pain. We do know that the mind–body connection, which I mentioned earlier, indicates a connection between levels of anxiety and the experience of pain.

If we can decrease your experience of anxiety and help you to learn how to help yourself relax and control your anxiety, then there can be a decrease in pain and an improvement in pain thresholds.

Working toward a goal, even if it's a small goal each day, will provide not only a focus for your day but also a sense of control—and control is something that you may have felt you had lost. Remember, you are on a journey, and this is one of the most worthwhile journeys of your life because it will directly contribute, on a daily basis, to the quality of your life.

The 11 Most Effective Self-Help Techniques

The following are the 11 most effective techniques to help lift mood, handle stressful situations, and cope with everyday anxiety.

Technique 1: Relaxation Breathing

Relaxation breathing is one of the simplest things you can learn to do. It really requires no training because you breathe naturally, but there's one catch and that's the secret here. What it does require is that you learn to focus on one specific thing during the exercise and nothing else. To begin, all you need to do is to find a quiet place, seat yourself comfortably, and proceed to engage in the exercise.

You'll be able to use it anywhere you wish, at any time in the future, and it will be yours. Once you get more comfortable with this exercise, you may begin to use it anytime, anywhere. You might be walking down the hallway in a building, down the street, waiting for a bus, going into an elevator, or anywhere you happen to be. Do it anywhere and it will be something that will relax you and it will call no attention to you. Should anyone note anything, all you need to say is, "Oh, I was sighing."

Remember, what I want you to do as this exercise begins is to concentrate first on the position of your feet and your toes. Think about where your feet are, where your toes are, and what they look like. Simple enough? Okay, let's begin!

The Exercise

Breathe in through your nose. Hold that breath as you count to five. Now breathe out through your mouth in a *whooshing* sound. Don't breathe in so fully that you become faint or that your muscles feel too tight. Just take comfortable, easy breaths. You're going to do this for a maximum of 5 times, but if that is too much when you first begin, it's okay to do it 2 or 3 times. It's really a matter of what is best for you, so you make the decision here, too.

Breathe in through your nose, hold it for a count of five, and then release your breath out through your mouth. *As you hold your breath for the count*, think about the position of your toes and your feet.

Now breathe in through your nose, hold it for a count of five. Think about where your knees are. Now breathe out through your mouth with that *whoosh* sound.

Each time you do this, think of a different part of your body. In other words, focus on a different part of your body, beginning with:

your toes and feet

your knees

your hips

your shoulders and arms

your hands

101

There you are. That's five different parts of your body on which to focus in a mental examination to see each feature. When you focus, in fact, you may want to superfocus. In other words, focus carefully on your toenails in your mind, look carefully at your feet, at your heels, at your toes, at your shoes. Really focus on them. The more vividly you can "see" them in your mind, the better. Don't allow yourself to be distracted.

The wonderful thing about this type of relaxation breathing is that it's perfectly natural and it's something that requires no practice at all. You breathe naturally, so this is just a way of turning that natural breathing into a wonderful, relaxing exercise.

But you're probably wondering how this could possibly do anything; it's only breathing, right? Well, it's not just breathing. When you do this simple exercise, you are causing a physiological change in your blood that has a relaxing effect. What is the change? You are balancing the carbon dioxide and oxygen in your blood.

Think about yawning when you're feeling tired and you'll understand that this is probably a natural reaction to trying to get more oxygen into your body to help you stay alert. You're taking in a large breath, probably several breaths, if you continue to yawn. Not only are you helping to balance your blood gases while using relaxation breathing, you're allowing yourself to take time out from the things that are stressing you or making you anxious. Just those few minutes concentrating on the position of your various body parts allows you the respite you need to break the stress cycle. It's like a mini "mind vacation," if you will. Everyone needs a vacation and here's one you may want to plan to have on a regular basis.

I have a feeling that you'll want to teach it to others once you find how well it works for you. In fact, it's okay because it's something you can share with others and you will be giving them a wonderful gift of relaxation and stress reduction. You may even want to share this with all your family members, because, as you are very much aware, your family is probably experiencing quite a bit of stress, too. A less stressed family is surely going to be a happier family.

As I said, this is something you will find helpful in any situation in your life, wherever you may find yourself. I can't think of a place where it might not be helpful.

Don't hesitate to use relaxation breathing several times a day, if you wish. Using it on a daily basis will help to release some of your built-up stress. It will give you more confidence because you will know that, going into a stressful situation, you now have a very effective tool for your own use. To use this tool, you need no prescription and no one's permission.

Relaxation breathing will also help you relax your muscles, so there is not only a decrease of stress and anxiety but also a decrease in muscle tension. As you know, muscle discomfort or pain is often related to levels of stress and anxiety. Anything that you can do to relax your muscles and decrease your anxiety is going to be beneficial to you in terms of any body discomfort you may have been experiencing. It can also be a helpful exercise to use if you have any stress associated with taking injectable medications; use it prior to an injection where muscle tension can be a problem. In this way, we can see that there are a whole host of benefits associated with simple breathing.

You may, in fact, want to teach it to any health care professionals who are working with you in order that they may use it with others. Now you are effectively sharing a therapeutic gift with them.

Along with relaxation breathing, you can also use progressive muscle relaxation exercises. These are simple and follow much the same course as you have just seen in relaxation breathing. Discussed next are the procedures on how you do this exercise.

Technique 2: Progressive Muscle Relaxation

With this exercise you will begin with your feet and progress up your body (from feet to head), repeating the same *tensing-and-releasing procedure* and thinking about what you're doing and nothing else:

1. Tense up the muscles of your feet for 5 seconds, then relax for 30 seconds.

2. Tense up your calves for 5 seconds, then relax for 30 seconds.

3. Now, your thighs and stomach for 5 seconds, and relax for 30 seconds.

4. Shoulders and chest for 5 seconds, and relax for 30 seconds.

5. Head and neck (not necessary if you have any discomfort in this area) for 5 seconds, and relax for 30 seconds.

The simple action of tensing and relaxing has a calming effect, and you will feel it almost immediately. It is, in fact, one of the most popular exercises currently being used in various rehab and medical settings.

The theory behind this type of tension- or anxiety-relieving technique goes back half a century. A physician, Edmund Jacobson, noticed that this type of flexing or tension on muscles, followed by relaxing resulted in a feeling of comfort. He theorized that it is impossible to have relaxed muscles and feel anxious at the same time. There is science behind this, and it is used in behavioral therapy today. Again, as in other forms of relaxation, you don't have to have a specific place to do this, and you can do it anywhere to give yourself a dose of relaxation.

Technique 3: Guided Imagery

Guided imagery is another very effective relaxation technique, and, in fact, along with relaxation breathing, it is something that you don't even need to learn. You've been doing some of this for much of your life in terms of daydreaming, but now we are going to put that skill to a slightly different use. I'll bet that you've done some of it while you were riding in a car, boarding a plane, or even listening to someone giving a rather boring speech.

Guided imagery involves mentally putting yourself in another place while your mind allows you to enjoy that moment without restriction. It's really similar to the distraction techniques dentists use when they are going to do some procedure where you might be a bit tense, say during a novacaine injection—they pull on your lip and tap on the gum and before you know it, it's done.

The Exercise

Once again, all you need to do is have a quiet, comfortable place where you can be by yourself for at least 10 to 15 minutes. If you'd like to do it for a bit longer, that's fine. Now, you need to think of a place where you once went or where you wish you could go. This should be a place that is both relaxing, enjoyable, and refreshing. Some people enjoy thinking about walking along a beautiful, white sandy beach with waves just coming up to the shore, looking out on the horizon. Other people prefer different scenes such as walking through a lovely meadow or an incredibly beautiful old library with carved ceiling and bookcases and a thick Persian rug on the floor. Wherever you feel you would be most comfortable is where you will place yourself now. You might even take to your computer, go to the National Geographic Web site, and download one of their beautiful wallpaper photos to provide a point of focus for you. Who said you couldn't go to Fiji?

To begin, you close your eyes. Use just a bit of your relaxation breathing, perhaps 2, 3, or 4 breaths, and instead of thinking about your toes, your knees, and your hips, think about that wonderful and peaceful place where you would like to be right now. Walk around that place and notice everything that there is to see. Take a look at what's under your feet; see what's to the right, to the left, or off in the distance. Look very carefully at the details of the place.

You'll be creating the scenarios here, so they can be as elaborate or as simple as you wish. You can use the same one each time or vary them. You will get the same result as long as you've chosen a relaxed, comfortable, and peaceful place where you can go in your mind.

Technique 4: Laughter and Humor

When was the last time you truly laughed out loud? How often do you find yourself laughing? If the answer to either of these is you can't remember or you don't laugh very often, now's the time to change all of that.

It's a fact that laughter is proven to have the ability to change heart rate, skin temperature, blood pressure, pulmonary ventilation, skeletal muscle activity, and brain activity, which may also have an effect on our overall sense of well-being. There is some belief in the research community that humor may actually have an important effect on stress chemicals and on what is called immunoenhancement. In other words, it may help bolster the immune system while it cuts back on the production of stress hormones such as cortisol.

Cortisol is a well-known stress-related hormone, which is often higher in the morning and may contribute to feelings of early morning distress. Although it serves an important purpose in our bodies, excessive amounts of cortisol have been shown in many studies over the past several decades to contribute to the breakdown of bodily tissues. This state has been compared to our bodies constantly being in a state of alarm. Anything that can be used to control this hormone and prevent it from reaching prolonged, harmful levels may be seen as useful. Here's where the wonder of laughter comes into the picture.

For the last 3 decades, medical schools and physicians, as well as others in the allied health care professions, have realized that laughter is really a therapeutic technique. Some medical schools, in fact, now have regularly scheduled seminars on the subject of laughter and humor, and it is used in treating individuals with a large variety of physical disorders from cancer, to pulmonary and cardiac disorders, Alzheimer's disease, stroke, and other disorders and diseases.

It's not a miracle cure, but laughter can contribute to important changes in your outlook, your mood, and even your immune system's functioning. How it can help your immune system help you is still not clear. As they say, the jury is still out for some investigators. Others have chosen to continue using this technique because they have found it does work, and for them and for many others as well as for the patients they treat, it has been a wonderful addition to their therapies.

As you may now know from psychoneuroimmunology, there is evidence to support the use of humor in healing. In fact, some studies have looked at the effects of laughter on physiological outcomes and how the use of humor in various illnesses as it is related to more favorable outcomes for patients. No one can doubt that lowering stress has an extremely beneficial effect on the immune system. Laughter, therefore, which is a wonderful safety valve for releasing stress, can also help the immune system.

Let's take a moment and just look at laughter in and of itself. What happens when you laugh? Sounds like a pretty basic and almost silly question but give it some thought. When you laugh, what are you doing? You are exercising muscles in your face, in your chest, in your stomach, and there is also a resulting change that takes place in your mood and in your outlook. When you laugh, to paraphrase a quote from Joseph Wolpe, a famous psychologist, "you cannot be tense or stressed and relaxed at the same time." Laughter relaxes you. If you weren't relaxed, you couldn't laugh.

The change in your mood may actually be caused by a change in those wonderful mood-elevating neurotransmitters in our brains. So laughter, in a way, might even be seen as a "medicine." In fact, it's one of the least expensive medicines you will ever need. The cost to you is zero. You don't need health insurance to get this medicine. All you need is a willingness to allow yourself to see the silliness, the humor, and the joy in the things in your life and in the people around you. You may even find it beneficial to laugh at yourself at times. You've heard the expression, "You're taking yourself too seriously." There's a great deal of truth in that sometimes.

Now, you may be saying that there isn't much joy in your life, but there is. You're going to change that way of thinking right now. What can you do? For one thing, you can begin to watch any type of humorous program, either on television or your computer, which makes you laugh. Here, you're the doctor because you decide what you should use as your humor treatment of choice. No one can tell you what you should watch, what will be fun for you, or what will make you laugh. You're the final authority here. You have absolute control. Doesn't that feel wonderful?

How about jokes? Don't know any? Okay, get busy on the computer and look up sites that deal with jokes or funny cartoons. There are some Web sites that have a joke of the day. If any of them appeal to you, bookmark the site, print out the joke or whimsical expression, and post it in a prominent spot in your home or in several places in your home, so that you will be sure to see it frequently. Yes, you're going to seed your home with jokes. It may not seem like a great decorating idea, but it sure is a good idea to raise your mood. Come to think of it, if you want to use it as a decoration, find ways to include the jokes anywhere in your home.

I knew a woman whose husband really needed to have his mood raised while he was at work during the day. He worked at a very stressful job, and his physician was concerned that his blood pressure was being affected by the work. She loved him and wanted to do anything she could to help in this serious situation. So what did this woman do? She prepared his lunch each day, and on top of his sandwich, she put a little note—a joke. He loved it and he looked forward to lunchtime, because it gave him not only a lunch break, but also a joke with every meal. He then began to share these jokes with his coworkers and soon everyone in his office was looking forward to his joke of the day. Sharing worked to change the office environment. So sharing jokes in your home can have a similarly good effect on your home environment.

Don't reserve humor as something you only do when you really need it. If I were writing a prescription, I would say "use humor prn," meaning use it whenever you wanted or needed it. I know I'm stretching the meaning of prn a little, but that's okay.

Whenever you feel you're having a problem coping, break that cycle of helplessness with a "time out" for pleasure. Turn on the TV, watch a movie, or do whatever will make you feel good. I've known college students who, before they went into an extremely important exam, watched cartoons because it helped alleviate the stress they were experiencing. We now know it's a good idea. When most of your therapies consist of sometimes uncomfortable treatments or medications or rather sterile things that you must do, laughter and humor are a welcome change. Use it and use it often. Patch Adams, the physician who brought humor into the hospital, was really right on this one.

Technique 5: Yoga

One of the things that many people who were interviewed for this book indicated that they used for relaxation was yoga. Yoga and bike riding were probably the two most popular methods of relaxation and stress reduction for both men and women. Remember, recent medical studies have indicated that yoga is a good option for people living with MS for relieving fatigue and reducing stress.

Sarah, a young professional living in a major city, said,

> I am very involved in yoga because I find it very helpful. I really would be an advocate for yoga for anyone and there are books that show how you can modify yoga exercises even if you're in a wheelchair. Yoga is all about not hurting you, and just helping you, so you can always modify yoga exercises.
>
> It starts with the breath that will help calm you down, will give you more oxygen and a better mood. You can do it in your own home, too. But, if you can get out, the social aspect of yoga classes can be very helpful. Also, it's harder to motivate yourself if you're going to exercise by yourself.

Moreover, yoga isn't only for women, much as some people may think. Men can benefit just as much from this gentle form of muscle exercise and relaxation. Roger, a retired businessman, when talking about his exercise routine, indicated that yoga is a part of it.

> I used to go to the Y. I've had an MS setback recently and I'm not as involved as before. Originally, I swam and my routine was that just about every morning I swam, used an exercise bike, and did yoga. I wouldn't do this every single day, but every other day. I was doing the yoga and or the biking in between. The yoga has proven to be very important to me, physically, because it includes stretching and aerobics with it.

Technique 6: Music

You may have heard the expression, "Music hath charms to soothe a savage beast, to soften rocks, or bend a knotted oak." Truer words were never spoken. The usefulness of music has been demonstrated for those with physical or psychological disorders.

Music has an incredible ability to soothe, comfort, or energize you. Today, thanks to many technological advances, you can have music wherever you go. There's music in your home, in your yard, in your car, as you shop in the grocery store, or right in your pocket or purse in the form of a small MP3 player. Make music a part of your daily life. If anyone you know has found a particular tune to be helpful, ask him or her to share it, and vice versa. Give yourself the gift of music and you will enjoy it forever.

We've seen how beneficial music can be for patients who have undergone operations that may have proven stressful. Studies have shown that patients who experienced soothing music, both before and during the procedure, had shorter recuperation times than patients who hadn't had this experience. Certainly, anyone with a chronic illness needs anything that can help their bodies heal or maintain their level of current health, and music appears to be helpful for this purpose, too.

Music has become a component of complementary and alternative medicine (CAM) and, while not seen as "mainstream medicine," is being reevaluated once again with the emphasis on the mind–body approach to treating the whole patient, not portions of the physical body. In one Canadian study, 70% of patients with MS used CAM to improve health and to manage symptoms, and most consumers reported positive results. One of the CAMs used was music therapy.

The results of a review of articles on the subject of music with patients with MS indicated that there were demonstrated improvements in self-acceptance, anxiety, and depression. As a result of this review, the researchers found music therapy to be of benefit for both psychosocial and emotional problems. Music therapy has even been found to be of great benefit to cancer patients with mood disturbances and one article noted that 37% of the patients had mood improvement, less postoperative pain and pain-related distress, and a reduced fear of treatments.

Record whatever music you find most soothing, and it's there for you whenever you want or need it. Much of the music that has been used in research on music therapy and its effects has been soothing classical music. Therefore, classical music might be a genre you would want to begin using and then, if you want, put in some upbeat tunes for energy boosts. There are soothing or uplifting contemporary instrumentals or even religious hymns or songs that can be just as useful. It's your music and, once again, you're the boss. Maestro, name your tune.

Technique 7: Exercise

Exercise is invaluable in fighting both depression and anxiety because it affects mood-regulating brain chemicals. New research has also indicated that there may be evidence that aerobic exercise promotes a brain-derived neurotropic (growth) factor and, therefore, can be a contributor to brain health.

Recent research on magnetic resonance imaging (MRI) scans of two groups of patients with MS, those who were physically fit and those who were less fit, showed important differences in the brain. Patients who engaged in aerobic fitness programs were seen as having a "protective effect on parts of the brain that are most affected by multiple sclerosis," according to a recent study completed by Dr. Prakash at Ohio State University. It was the conclusion of that small study that more physically fit patients did better on tests of cognition, which depended on processing speed, a measure of concentrating and short-term memory, and is most closely associated with attention span. It is also a measure of the ability to remember instructions and complete tasks in a timely manner. Who thought exercise could improve your memory or concentration? It's a wonderful new finding.

Minding your body is an effective means of improving your mind and there is a powerful link between the two, according to psychologist Dr. Christopher Hertzog of the Georgia Institute of Technology. Hertzog and his associates reviewed the literature on physical exercise and memory. The team concluded that it appeared to have a significant effect on memory maintenance and even in reducing the odds for experiencing dementia. It didn't matter at what age the participants in the studies began their physical regimes, so beginning to exercise in midlife is just as valuable as beginning to exercise earlier. Exercise is bound to benefit the person no matter when he or she begins to include this in daily routines.

A 2006 study sought to see whether the brain responded physically to exercise. The researchers concluded that "relatively short exercise interventions can begin to restore some of the losses in brain volume associated with normal aging." The volunteers in the study were all between the ages of 60 and 79 years and participated in a 6-month fitness program.

Just walking can improve cognition in older adults, according to a large study of 5,925 women older than 65. One totally unexpected result that came out of the study was that the distance walked, regardless of the pace of walking, mattered more for limiting cognitive decline. So, if you're a slow walker, that's not going to matter; just walk.

Another large, multiyear study of 16,466 nurses older than the age of 70 tracked various physical activities in which they engaged. The activities included running, jogging, walking, hiking, racket sports, swimming, bicycling, and aerobic dancing. There was a positive relationship between the energy they expended and the cognitive benefit. In this study, there was a slightly different result, albeit a favorable benefit just the same, of how much energy was expended, unlike the walking study. Regardless of the slightly different conclusions, the result is incontrovertible—exercise is good for the brain and the mind.

Reading these research results, you may be asking yourself how this is going to benefit you since you may not be a senior citizen and you do have a chronic medical illness. You may even feel I'm treating this more like a course than a book meant to help you meet the challenges of MS as it relates to depression, anxiety, and cognition. The material is presented to provide something I consider impressive as it relates to physical exercise, no matter your age or your medical problems. The brain responds and it responds well to what you do physically.

I haven't tracked the studies (although they do exist) that look at wheelchair athletes but I would suspect that their willingness to maintain themselves in sports has reaped truly remarkable returns in life satisfaction. I would venture so far as to say that they probably experience better cognitive functions than those who do not engage in sports and that their level of anxiety, depression, and pain are probably lower, too.

I did see one 1990 study that indicated these "athletes scored significantly better than nonathletes on the mood state of depression." A 2009 CNN Health feature highlighted rugby wheelchair athletes who engage in this full-contact sport. Therefore, your MS doesn't necessarily disqualify you from expanding your physical horizons.

With MS, it may be difficult for you to even consider that you might be able to exercise in some form. You may feel you don't have the energy, you don't have the will, or you don't have the motivation that are required for any type of exercise. Although some of these definitely play a role, exercise can still be a part of your routine and your ongoing efforts to push away the depression and the anxiety, as well as the stress you may feel on a daily basis. It can actually *increase your energy level, give you motivation,* and *diminish the feeling of fatigue* that comes with MS or the depression that can accompany it. Is it worth a try? Of course it is!

As you would with any effort to bring about change in your life, and exercising may be a change for you, remember to be realistic about setbacks. You will have them and that doesn't mean all is lost. It just means you've had a minor detour and you need to get back on track and do what you need. Using it as an excuse to avoid trying exercise again isn't an option if you truly want to take charge of your physical condition as much as possible.

Psychologists talk about relapse prevention when they investigate change programs, and exercise has to have a prevention component. The element, of course, is knowing that it's going to happen, not "if" it happens. It will, but you'll know that in advance and push on despite it.

Keep in mind that depression, too, is going to be holding you back, and that depression will fight very hard to keep you from being motivated. But the first step that you take toward taking charge of your life, and any exercise you wish to engage in, is going to be the most important step you can take toward hitting back at depression. Depression is the enemy. Don't let it take you prisoner.

Some of the most exciting news of all about exercise has to do with potential repair of the brain. Exercise has been found to aid in the production of new nerve connection and brain volume as I mentioned earlier, and, possibly, nerve cells themselves. One interesting study of just what activities might add to these brain connections centered on juggling. The researcher, Dr. Heidi Johansen-Berg of the University of Oxford, as quoted in the media, said that, "We tend to think of the brain as being static, or even beginning to degenerate, once we reach adulthood. In fact, we find the structure of the brain is ripe for change. We've shown that it is possible for the brain to condition its own wiring to operate more efficiently."

In her research study, she had volunteers attend a class to learn to juggle once weekly and then train on their own for 30 minutes daily for 6 weeks. The research team performed prestudy and poststudy MRI scans of participants' brains to provide physical evidence of any improvement on nerve growth.

Changes were noted in the white matter areas of the brain (the material that carries information from nerve cell to nerve cell) that were linked to reaching, grasping, and peripheral vision. It didn't matter how proficient study participants had become at juggling, just that they continued to practice juggling daily. Dr. Johansen-Berg didn't recommend that people learn juggling so much as that they do some form of physical or mental exercise. Crossword puzzles or walking, she suggested, would also be good ideas. Juggling had been selected for this study simply because it was a new skill that the study participants did not possess and that they had to learn for the study. In this way, they countered any influence of prior learning.

Incredibly, in the past decade, we've seen that exercise has benefits we never dreamed of. The benefits aren't just limited to maintaining muscle tone or balance; it also tones and builds our brains. What type of exercise you do is best determined by you and your physician. Not everyone is going to want to go out and learn to juggle.

Sometimes simple things, such as tai chi (also called tai chi chuan), are intended to be a nonstrenuous series of planned slow movements and balance exercises. Some people have characterized it as "meditation in motion." In this form, the exercises are variations of rhythmic patterns coordinated with breathing. The goal is a calming action. Much like mindfulness, tai chi requires that you be "in the moment" as you do the graceful moves, and it is exercise, rather than strength, that is your target.

One thing you will find interesting is that exercise of any kind can have a beneficial effect on your endorphins, those brain substances that are called the "feel good" neurotransmitters. It's something that keeps runners running because they get that boost called the "runner's high" from them. So, it's a mood elevator, and who doesn't want that?

Some forms of tai chi can be more strenuous or fast paced than others, but there are forms that are intended for anyone, requiring some physical activity, but done in an enjoyable manner. Specific programs have been developed for persons older than 50, so this is exercise really geared to all ages, not just the younger, more flexible individuals. Do you need an outfit? Is there any equipment required? None that I know of. You only need to wear clothing that is loose and comfortable.

The benefits of this exercise regime, according to some preliminary research, are the following:

- Reduced anxiety and depression;
- Improved balance, flexibility, and muscle strength;
- Lowered blood pressure;
- Relief of chronic pain;
- Improved quality of sleep;
- Increased energy, endurance, and agility; and
- A general feeling of overall wellness

Tai chi, as you can see, measures up very well with several of the other forms of self-help techniques that we've mentioned.

The proper physical form is all-important in this exercise and that comes with practice, so don't expect to accomplish everything in one session. It is recommended that you work with an experienced instructor who understands the limitations of age and illness when people perform the tai chi moves. Overly vigorous moves can strain muscles, as has been seen in first-time tai chi practitioners. The recommendation is usually that you join a class and stick with it at the same time, same place each week so that you make it a stable part of your routine. Again, the social and supportive elements of the tai chi group, as well as the commitment to attending, are added benefits.

Other exercises may be as simple as walking in place, doing arm or leg lifts or anything that will help you feel more mobile and capable. *Walking in place* is also something that can be done anywhere. So do it while you're waiting for an elevator, standing in line at the supermarket, or waiting for a bus. Do it anywhere and keep putting those minutes down on your exercise chart (Appendix C).

In your home, you can walk in place for just 5 minutes in the morning when you get up. It's 5 minutes more exercise than you would have had, so pat yourself on the back and keep up the good work. Feeling that this would be boring? Okay, turn on the TV, watch the weather report (usually only 3–4 minutes), and do the walking in a "mindless" fashion as you watch and listen to the meteorologist. You will have met your goal faster than you thought. In addition, the nice part about this is that you can do it with no concerns about the actual weather outside. What a bonus!

If you want to get more out of walking in place, gently swing your arms as you walk. Mark it down on your exercise form and put the chart on your fridge. It's a way to get started and that's all you have to do now: get started doing something.

As you feel more comfortable and build up your stamina, you can try to do 10 minutes of walking, but you might want to keep it at 5 minutes so you don't tire yourself. Of course, talk to your physician or rehab specialist about how much walking in place you can do.

Interestingly, music and singing can also be used in a form of exercise, not in the dance mode, but in an exercise for respiratory muscle strength. Music emphasizes diaphragmatic breathing and coordination of breath and speech, and it may be of benefit to some people with MS.

Search out groups in your area that specialize in helping people with MS in either personal or group participation in an exercise program. Group exercise adds a dimension of socialization and motivation to keep going, which exercising alone doesn't offer. It is very important that whoever is responsible for the group be fully aware of MS, its symptoms, and limitations.

National MS organizations may be of help in finding local exercise groups in your area. If there isn't a group currently, perhaps you have found something where you can now make a contribution to both your own health and that of your neighbors as well. Ever think of starting an MS exercise group, perhaps through a local hospital or social service group in your area? Doing so can provide you with a sense of purpose, boost your self-esteem, and make something wonderful available in your area. Give it some thought. No, I'm not trying to pressure you. I'm just providing food for thought.

Swimming has been seen as an effective form of exercise, and Roger chooses swimming as one of his exercise routines. The routine he had managed to carve out for himself didn't work out as well as he had hoped because his MS began to cause his physical skills to falter. "I have had several bouts that have taken me out of the swimming game. When a lifeguard is pacing the edge of the pool with his life-saving equipment as you're swimming, it's not a very good feeling. Quite honestly, my feet were just dangling beneath me, and I was doing the swimming with my arms more than anything else. So I had pushed as far as I could push it at the time. Today, I am much better."

A regime of endurance training with weights is in Roger's plan as is his maintaining his resolve knowing that "with each and every MS flare up, I'm starting over again." As he said, "Hope is the energy that drives me. It's very important."

Anna, who you met in an earlier chapter, has continued her at-home exercise. She knows that she can't do as much as she would like, but she's determined to continue doing whatever she can on her stationary bicycle. Her difficulty is almost entirely with her legs and she has devised a method to keep them moving with the help of her hands and arms pulling on her pants. She has not given up even though her symptoms have worsened later in life.

One of the problems that people indicate regarding exercise is that they see it as something that has to be done outside the home and, often, the weather is a major consideration. Technology, however, is on our side. While I don't normally recommend specific exercise equipment, I am going to recommend something now. I've seen from my own experience and that of others that the Nintendo console known as the Wii Fit Plus offers a wide variety of exercise routines, which can be fit into just about anyone's daily schedule. The routines include yoga, jogging, a series of balance exercises, and several exercises aimed at physical coordination, judgment, and reaction time.

You can tailor your routine to whatever fits your need best and it will keep track of your performance, the number of calories you burn, and one additional important measure: your body mass index (BMI). The BMI is an important measure of overall healthy weight.

If you'd like to calculate your BMI on your own without doing any actual math, there is a Web site from the National Institutes of Health (http://www.nhlbisupport.com/bmi/) that will do the calculation for you, just enter your height and weight. There's also a chart, which indicates to you how you're doing in terms of maintaining a healthy BMI. Here's how they note them:

BMI Categories:

- Underweight = <18.5
- Normal weight = 18.5–24.9
- Overweight = 25–29.9
- Obesity = BMI of 30 or greater

You can set your goal for your exercise routine and this goal can be adjusted as needed, so flexibility is built into the program. The program even offers encouragement, and I believe it is a great way to ensure that you do have some daily exercise. You can build up your endurance and tone your muscles, too.

Additionally, you can do it by yourself, in a group, or with just one other person. You don't need to worry about weather, getting to a class on time, or ever missing your exercise because of other commitments or appointments. You can do it in the middle of the night if you want. How good is that?

When you think of exercise, one thing that comes to mind is the chronic feeling of fatigue. Physical activity and its relationship to fatigue and depression in individuals with MS have been addressed in research studies. One study that included 292 people with MS found that physical activity resulted in a greater sense of self-efficacy, which, in turn, led to a decrease in feelings of fatigue and depression. The researchers believed people living with MS developed a greater sense of mastery through physical exercise and that this played a part in decreasing their depression, which had been adding a greater sense of fatigue. Therefore, once again, we see how this cycle of depression, fatigue, and exercise works.

Beginning to exercise breaks the cycle and clears the way for enhanced physical activity and improved mood. It's in your hands and you do have power to change things in a significant way by doing several simple things on a daily basis. You don't have to overextend yourself, but you do have to try each day, just a bit, to work in your own best interest and toward your own goal. Be your own coach, don't overly tire yourself, but don't be ready to stop too quickly. Of course, check with your doctor before beginning any type of exercise routine.

Gerald, One Outstanding Example of How Exercise Works

Although this section is devoted exclusively to self-help techniques, there is one person whose story must be added right here in the exercise section because he stands out as a shining example of what can be done with, as he said, "a little OCD" as it relates to his illness. Unique in the results he has achieved, we present him not as typical of what can be accomplished, but as someone who decided to seek out solutions for himself.

When he was in his late 50s, Gerald noticed that one leg dragged after he finished his ride on an exercise bike. There were other symptoms, too. He experienced fatigue, uncharacteristic bumping into furniture, and balance problems. Once the diagnosis was made of progressive primary MS 20 years ago, Gerald decided that he would use his professional skills to tackle it as a research question that he would seek to answer. The Internet was in its infancy, but it did provide some research and he used this along with lots of library trips and a local research librarian. The literature he reviewed pointed to consideration of diet and exercise, both of which he incorporated into his revised lifestyle.

In an early evening interview, Gerald told me, "Fifteen to 20 years ago, they told you not to exercise and there's a good reason for it. The core temperature goes up like a degree or two." Remember what Dr. Gold said about those really being "pseudoexacerbations"? But, as Gerald pointed out, exercise has been the most beneficial thing he has done for himself. In fact, he has proven to be such a stellar example of self-help in MS therapy that, "My neurologist writes on his prescription pad, 'Do what Gerald does' and gives it to MS patients."

His workplace was attuned to the benefits of exercise for everyone and had a fitness center installed for its employees. As he said,

> Fortunately, I was able to use the fitness [center] at work and I used to ride a stationary bike 10 miles and I used to walk around the track to cool off and I noticed that one leg would drag a little. I discounted it because I thought it was because I was getting a little bit older. By the time I took a shower I was back to normal. As time went on, I found I was dragging my foot even after a shower.

The problems persisted and Gerald knew something was wrong; it wasn't just normal aging. "I went to see my family physician and he said everything was perfect but I went to see a neurologist. He did an MRI and I got the diagnosis of primary progressive MS and I almost couldn't ride the bike; I couldn't do anything."

He found himself incredibly fatigued as he tried to do his normal work at his job.

> I was weak as a kitten and couldn't do anything. My family physician told me he didn't know anything about MS but he gave me some sage advice and it was, "Work on your overall

wellness." So, the first thing that came to my mind was diet. The fitness center at work had a dietician who helped find some research on diet, which wasn't helpful because I was already doing some of the things that came up in the search. However, my rule was "try anything as long as it's inexpensive and safe." I found another man on the Internet who had a son who had MS and we teamed up doing research in the existing literature.

After reviewing voluminous amounts of research, Gerald knew what he had to do. "I decided that I wanted to start an exercise program. By that time I had retired because I was struggling with draining fatigue and it was just killing me. Once I retired, I was able to devote my full time to exercise and research."

Everything he did, Gerald did slowly and in moderation. "I started walking in the pool and I did that for about 2 years. Then I decided to see if I could swim for 15 minutes and I did that. I saw a friend swimming with a snorkel and I thought that was a great idea because you don't have to worry about breathing." He found it helped with his focus on other actions with his body in the water. "I could concentrate on other things and I bought fins because I wanted to put more load on my legs to get more strength."

As the snorkel and fins worked out well, he began increasing his time in the pool. "The next thing I knew, I was swimming an hour after many months. My mantra was, 'Do everything very slowly.' So, I bought a weight machine and a stationary bike that I use at home. Three times a week I'd go to the fitness center and swim. The next thing I knew, I was swimming 2 hours at a time."

Although he had increased his swim time, "there was still that need to concentrate with all my neurons to say 'kick' and it was an incredible task. Then, I don't know how much time passed, I realized I wasn't thinking about kicking. I wondered if I could do the same thing with walking." This led to the next phase of his self-imposed program.

"So I began to walk around the house, and one day I was able to walk once around the track at the fitness center. It's 14 laps for a mile and the trainer started watching me and he said, 'Hey, you need to learn how to walk.' Walking is a very complicated task. It's electrical, it's mechanical, and a combination of all the things that happen in the body. They had to teach me how to walk."

"They asked why I was making a clenched fist. I didn't know I was doing it. They told me not to do it because that gets translated into your neck and it puts extra stress into your body." The simple act of walking turned into another action that required remediation.

Gerald remembers, "They would walk with me and correct me as I walked. So, I was able to do one lap by myself and after a few months I asked a friend to walk with me around the track to see if I could walk and talk at the same time. Couldn't do it. My brain just couldn't handle it, and the trainer told me to just look at the white line and not to look anywhere else. The problem was that I was getting distracted by all the fancy exercise equipment inside the track area."

The trainers kept working with Gerald for years. His determination would seem astonishing, but he admits he did have days that he struggled to get himself going. But he never gave up and he always added to his program.

"Next, I decided that I had to be able to jog. The first time I started to jog, I did 10 steps. Next time, it was 70 steps. Eventually, I was able to jog once around the track and then one-quarter mile. Jogging was really a personal challenge and once I accomplished it, I went back to walking. After a little over 5 years, I was able to walk 2 miles."

His routine is invariable. "Three days a week I go to the fitness center for swimming and walking, 2 days at home riding a stationary bike for 15 to 20 miles and doing weight lifting. I wanted to try to cover all the exercises that I could, and I do full body exercises over different days."

"On my 70th birthday, I got a bug in my head that I was going to swim 3 hours and I did it. I couldn't believe it. Now, for my 75th birthday I'm training for a 3-hour swim again. I had been doing 2-hour swims until I got an infection and a violent reaction to an antibiotic, and I'm back to 1 hour again."

Gerald's neurologist makes it a point to call him because Gerald doesn't have regular appointments. "I got into an argument with my neurologist who calls me and says he hasn't seen me as a patient for 3 years and wants me to come to his office. I don't ever go to see him because all we do is shake hands, say hello and that's it. He told me that what I'm doing is helpful, and I keep telling him that he doesn't know that. I tell him that we have to be scientific about this and I'm only one data point. I would, however, like to believe it's helping."

"If someone proves to me, beyond the shadow of a doubt, that what I'm doing is of no value in MS, I wouldn't change a thing." In fact, Gerald admits that if he doesn't exercise he feels as though he were being punished and his diet, which consists essentially of fruits, vegetables, nuts, fish, chicken, bread, and a variety of vitamins, was to his liking.

The results appear to be promising. "I've had a few MRIs and they found there's no change in my brain since I started my program. My neurologist has noticed no progression in my MS over the past 8 years. On the Expanded Disability Status Scale, which is an objective measure of your walking by a physician who determines how you're doing, I went from 4 to 1, which was impressive."

What does he do to keep himself going and to keep exercising? "Some days aren't so good for me, but everyone has days like that. It's my attitude and if I don't feel well, I decide I'll do it tomorrow. I say, 'Well, I don't have to do this at all.' You'd be amazed how often this happens and what you think is important is not that important at that moment. I push forward and I always feel better after I do my exercises. I feel like a new person."

On days when he's feeling a bit reluctant to engage in his program, he persists. "When I go to the fitness center, I tell myself that I'm only going to swim for 15 minutes, then I do 15 and then I decide I can do another 15. The next thing I know, I've done an hour or 2 hours. I do the same thing with weight lifting." It's this gradual introduction to the exercises that engages him.

Although most people might prefer group activity to keep them motivated, Gerald prefers a more solitary approach to most of it.

> I do all of this by myself, not in a group because I'm the only one home during the day. I swim by myself but walk with another man and then, after our walk, we have a discussion. This keeps our brain exercised. Sometimes we talk about books or things in the news, European news, or any topic that comes to mind. I try to do the best I can. I still have MS and the chances of it disappearing are slim, but I'm in my 70s and I think I'm doing much better than most men my age. Attitude is important. How do I keep my attitude positive? I just say that tomorrow's another day and today I'm going to do the best I can.

What is a typical day for this 70-something man?

> The way I start my day is that I get up between 6 and 7, read the newspaper while I'm having breakfast, check my email, look at MS research on the Internet, then I go to the fitness center or to the basement to do my exercise. I go to class at 1 or 2 [PM] and I also teach a class. Afterward, when I come home, I check my e-mail again and I read. I have always liked reading and I read everything from newspapers, magazines, books and the Internet. It's a very full day and I love it.

Gerald and a group of men in the classes he takes discovered that, over the summer when there were no classes, they could form their own group. They meet for lunch twice a week and then have a book review session afterward. Sometimes, they have speakers come to their group. It's another part of his creativity that he has found serves him well.

Technique 8: Biofeedback

While biofeedback may not seem like a self-help technique, it really is. However, you will need a bit of equipment, if you want to use it on your own. Biofeedback is useful for everything from migraine headache to muscle pains, gastric distress, high blood pressure, sleep disorders, anxiety, and a whole host of other disorders. It is something that is generally done in the office of a certified biofeedback clinician, but they do have small pieces of equipment that can be used in the home once you've been trained by a clinician. I know it sounds like something involved or technical, but it's pretty simple stuff. I did, in fact, have training in biofeedback, so I am very familiar with it and what it can do.

Generally, it involves little more than listening to a relaxation tape, and having a small electrode taped to one finger. When I say "electrode," I know that sounds like it might be painful, but it's not. It's nothing more than a small contact that communicates with a machine and feeds information such as your heart rate or whether or not you are sweating back to that machine. You've probably had this type of equipment used in hospitals where they now check your body temperature or blood flow to your fingers via one of these little contacts. There is no possibility of shock involved, trust me.

Sessions can take from 15 to 30 minutes, and during that time you will be using some relaxation breathing and guided imagery. As you do, you may either see a monitor that will show you your heart rate or skin temperature or a musical or other tone will be played. All of this is the "feedback" portion of the therapy.

What you are receiving is information about how well your body is learning to relax even though you are unaware that you are actively causing these changes. After a number of sessions, you will be able to lower your blood pressure, change some aspects of body temperature, if that is desirable, and your heart rate. You will do this, in fact, almost without being aware that you are doing it. That's the wonder of biofeedback. It's almost effortless. Some biofeedback equipment can be used to monitor muscles that are involved in back pain and to see how effectively these muscles can be brought under control and taught to relax.

You usually receive the confirmation that you are now controlling some body function by a change in the tone that is played. So, there may be a constant humming sound and then a beep when you get the body control you seek. Again, that's the feedback.

After you've mastered the techniques, you will be able to use them to help yourself reduce your stress and anxiety by yourself. I mention temperature changes as an important skill that biofeedback can teach because we have seen great benefit in persons who have problems with circulation in their hands (known as Raynaud's syndrome and is often found, too, in other individuals without this syndrome but who suffer from stress).

We know that stress causes blood to leave the hands and feet and make its way to the core of the body. This is in preparation for what is known as the "fight or flight" fear reaction, and it's a hallmark of stress. The temperature in your fingers can be a good indicator of how stressed you are, so being able to measure changes in finger temperature can serve as a good stress index for you. Some devices that do this are simple little business cards with a temperature-sensitive patch on them. Placing your finger on the patch for a few seconds will give you a reading. Once you have that, you can begin to do some of the relaxation techniques you've learned in the biofeedback sessions.

Technique 9: Positive Self-Talk and Arguing

Remember when people thought that talking to yourself meant you had a serious mental problem? Then we began to see athletes, particularly tennis players, not only talking to themselves, but shouting at themselves, much like a coach, on the tennis court. They were doing a very smart thing, even though they may not have known it or may have stumbled on it as a way to vent their frustration. Self-talk works and it works well. So, let's take a look at what you might call "self-coaching."

What happens when you speak out loud to encourage yourself, push yourself, or offer some words of consolation? For one thing, you are using major portions of your brain power, and your brain is "listening" to what you're saying. Yes, it's actively listening to you.

In order to say something out loud, you have to first form the thought (your brain thinking centers), then you have to form speech (the brain speech centers), next you have to vocalize it (muscle centers to pull the vocal cords, tongue, facial, and mouth muscles), and it's heard by your ears (your brain's speech detection centers). So, look at how much of your brain power is used in just forming the self-talk you use and how many muscle groups are engaged. And, don't forget, there's something called "muscle memory" involved here. We'll talk about that a bit later.

It's amazing how involved the mind gets in this. Once the ears hear something, the rest of the brain jumps into action and has to process it to make sense of what was heard. In this final action, we get through to the real centers that matter where the brain "hears" this as something that "makes sense." How it does all of this is a miracle of nature.

If you're thinking that someone told you that an important memory center in your brain has suffered injury, keep in mind the story of one man who is still teaching scientists about memory and the brain: Kim Peek. He was born with serious problems in his nervous system development, and he was missing a vital connection, the corpus callosum, a tissue connection between the two halves or hemispheres of his brain. Despite this, he developed the most incredible memory ever recorded and read 12,000 books during his lifetime, using each eye independently to scan the pages of books. This truly incredible man points to the fact that the brain uses many pathways for memory, not just the ones about which we currently know. Mother Nature still amazes us with her magic.

So, what do you say to yourself in this self-talk? Remember, it's got to be positive, no beating yourself up here, no rehashing what went wrong before or how you may not have done something or didn't do it "correctly." There's no reason to go over the past. Right now, it's all future focused and results oriented. It's your call again.

Suggestions:

1. Okay, we can do this. (Repeat it several times as you do the action.)

2. That's okay, not everything is going to work out the first time, so let's think of another way to do it.

3. The *Little Engine That Could* has nothing on me, so let's keep on and do it.

   One illustration of incredible determination in the face of seemingly unwinnable odds was shown by Dr. Milton Erickson, a psychiatrist who had postpolio syndrome as an adult and was paralyzed and wheelchair bound. He had polio as a teenager and decided he wasn't going to give up, and each day he worked by looking at his small "pinky" finger and trying to get it to move. In time, he succeeded and then proceeded to work on other fingers, his hand and, gradually, his upper body. The result of all his effort was that he could walk with a cane, went to medical school, and then had a relapse that meant that, even though he couldn't walk any longer, he perfected a form of hypnosis, based on individual stories or metaphors, which helped people make dramatic changes in their lives.

4. Just give yourself some time. It's okay. Relax and give yourself a break now.

5. Slow down, you don't have to do it all at once. It's okay to do it a bit slower.

A word on muscle memory: This is a relatively new area that is being explored by psychologists and medical professionals and even in training. Muscle memory is something that professional and amateur athletes have been utilizing in their training to enhance their performances in their individual sports. But I believe it has some use here, too.

Once you train yourself to use positive self-talk, you've actually trained yourself to respond, in terms of your vocal chords and facial muscles, to pull up that memory and therefore, it becomes something you do more naturally. You don't have to think about doing it anymore because you'll begin to do it almost as a reflex. It could be called a form of "mental karate" because, in that sport, most of the action depends on hours of rigorous exercise routines where you learn to respond automatically, without thinking. Your automatic actions here are going to be composed of giving yourself encouragement and stressing the positive things you've done.

How does it apply here? Someone takes an action (let's say in your case it's you making a negative self-comment) and you respond with the appropriate counteraction (positive self-talk). Do it enough times and it becomes second nature. You can also use a form of self-talk with mental imagery or mental rehearsal if you are having a particular problem with something. Visualize yourself in the situation in your mind, go over the possible ways to handle it, and then "watch" yourself perform it. Everyone rehearses and so should you.

Dr. Martin Seligman, a well-known psychologist and advocate of positive psychology, advises that you not only use positive self-talk but that you also learn to argue with yourself. Argue? Don't you have enough people in your life arguing with you as it is? The answer is "no," because here you're going to use this "arguing" for a very different reason—to get at the truth of the current problem and evaluate it more fully. Seligman doesn't intend for there to be any emotion in this arguing; it's more like a questioning discussion with yourself or use of what is called the Socratic Method, which is used in law schools.

So, how do you argue and what should you do to get started? First, let me interject something that I think is relevant. Another famous psychologist, Dr. Julian Rotter, speculated about our expectancies regarding our lives. He believed that we maintain a certain "locus of control" in our beliefs about ourselves, and from this we form the reasons or beliefs about why things happen to us. In other words, are we truly the masters of our fate or does someone else control it? If we are what Rotter called "internals," we believe we are at fault when things happen to us and we can see this as:

1. I didn't try hard enough.
2. I didn't have the ability.

If you believe that it's not you that brought the problem into your life, but someone or something in your life, you believe in less or no personal control and you are an "external" and you see it as:

1. They don't like me or don't want me to succeed.
2. They made it too hard for me to succeed.

The first approach is, by far, the better one because it conveys a sense of ownership over your life and what happens to you and that's going to benefit you. If you find that you're using the second one quite a bit, then you have some arguing to do with yourself, and that's where Seligman's method can be helpful.

One word of caution is advisable here. Not everyone in every situation is going to be either internal or external. Sometimes there will be switches, but you may find that the scales are tipping more toward one end than the other and there are some adjustments that need to be made.

According to Seligman, your "arguing" should include:

1. Looking for evidence to support or dispute your beliefs;

2. Searching for alternative reasons why something happened;

3. Asking yourself what the implications are if you think this way. (Are you cultivating a "Chicken Little" view of the world? You may be catastrophizing and only seeing things in a dire light); and

4. Identifying how useful is it for you to think this way. Does it work toward your advantage or disadvantage? Are you getting any particular gain from this or is it adding to your burden?

Put this type of thinking/questioning into action right away and begin to use it on anything that has happened to you in the past week. If you want, begin to make a list of things and then go over each item on the list to see where you stand. How do your expectations stand up in the light of this type of "arguing?"

Actually, engaging in this type of arguing is using a technique that is very similar to what cognitive psychologists use in psychotherapy. The whole premise is to get you to throw out the automatic thoughts and the quick slips into catastrophizing, and to more properly attribute actions to the real world. This is truly changing your thinking around. Once you begin to practice arguing, you may find that you are more prone to one or the other type of thinking than you ever thought.

One additional word of advice here on how to phrase questions you may want to pose to someone or even to yourself: The way to keep a conversation of any kind going is never, never to ask what we call closed-ended questions. These are questions that someone can easily answer with a simple "yes" or a "no." So, while you're practicing your self-talk here, try to use open-ended questions such as "*What was it that caused you to think that way?*" or "*Now what might you do here to get this resolved?*" These are both good ways to begin searching for answers that will help you get to where you need to go. Additional note here: remember to smile when you ask these questions. It's the easiest way to smooth any conversation, so practice using it, even if you have to stand in front of a mirror to do it.

Please, whenever you feel like beating yourself up, pull back for a few minutes and take a fresh view of the situation. If you're feeling you've done something that wasn't too smart, don't see yourself as "stupid." Everyone makes mistakes and we can all learn from them.

No one *always* has "the right answer" for everything and none of us were born with an ingrained manual that contains all the instructions we will ever need and all the answers for all the questions we will ever have asked of us. Use each of these situations to your advantage. Live in hope and let that be your guiding star each day and through each evening. Remember, the stars are out during the daytime but you can't see them because the sun outshines them. Hope is there, too, and just like the stars, you may not see it, but it's there if you look for it and believe that it is there.

Technique 10: Journaling

I think there should be a new proverb and it should be, "*Writing is for relief.*" I'm talking, of course, about journaling and its advantages. Roger is a big proponent of journaling, which he actually began in his youth. As he told me when we talked, "Mind your thoughts; mind what's going on in your head, and what you're thinking. Anxiety, in my case, in my opinion, and my experience is what's bothering me.

"If I were writing this book, I would try to clarify whether anxiety is something that is going on in the mind and causing the problem. Are we talking negatively to ourselves or is this something physical that is actually going on in the body?" He has gotten into the habit of intelligently questioning himself.

Roger knows how to practice what he preaches and he's humble about it. "I'm not so sure that I'm a perfect example. I find writing helps me a lot because I can write my thoughts down and as I'm writing I can stay in tune with what I'm saying to myself and others. I write to myself, nobody has to read it. I keep a journal where I express myself."

So, is Roger rehearsing in a way? I think so and he's engaging in self-talk prior to any interactions so that he has an opportunity to look at something from other perspectives than the one that might come immediately to mind. He's double-checking things.

He might be angry or,

I might be frustrated, but I might be truly positive, too. It's just a way for me to vent. Then I can review what I've written to make sure that what I express in writing is really what I intend to express. Am I really saying accurately what I'm feeling? Once I've been able to do that, then I can clearly communicate with others about what I'm feeling. When I do that, I feel better about myself and I feel we can go on with our relationship as it has always been.

Journaling is a means to vent without observation, to question without concern, and to be solution-oriented.

For me, journaling works. Today, I find that journaling is as important as my daily exercise. This mental exercise that I'm going through is very important. Analyzing what has been written helps me to stay positive, but it also allows me to check my thoughts. When I think I'm feeling crummy, do I always feel crummy? If I remove that word *always*, it becomes, "I feel crummy today." I don't *always* feel crummy.

He's managed to turn this type of situation around so that he can more accurately, as he indicated, see how he feels and know that it's not as bad as it first seemed. Roger does not catastrophize; he looks for solutions. Doesn't it also sound like Roger is, without knowing it, using that "arguing" we just indicated in the last tip? Roger has also started writing an Internet blog to help others see that they are not alone and to make his struggle become part of their increasing knowledge about MS and how it affects individuals. He's willing to reveal his struggle in order to provide examples of ways for individuals with MS to learn how to fight against it.

Technique 11: Meditation and Mindfulness

A lot has been written about meditation and its benefits, and, in fact, we do know that many outpatient programs in hospitals and rehab centers have included a meditation component in their programs.

Although most people refer to this as meditation, there is a new term that is being used now and it is *mindfulness meditation*. It is also being referred to as *integrative medicine* because it affects a wide range of stress, pain, and chronic diseases. Numerous research studies have shown meditation to be a potent endeavor in terms of brain activity and physical changes with regard to antibody production. Therefore, this would appear to be something that you would want to incorporate into your weekly schedule, if possible.

Mindfulness has been shown to lower levels of the stress hormone, cortisol, and may have a positive effect of increased motivation for important lifestyle change. It can reduce depression, anxiety, and provide an increased ability to tolerate and possibly decrease the need for certain types of anxiolytic or pain medications. There has also been improved adherence to medical treatments. As you can see, it has wide-ranging, positive effects even though it would appear to be quite a simple thing to do.

Mindfulness has been seen as effective in all of the following:

1. Decreased pain perception;
2. Increased tolerance of pain;
3. Reduced stress, anxiety, and depression—all good things;
4. Potential decrease in need for pain medications via anxiety reduction;
5. Change in ability regarding making medical treatment decisions because of improved sense of self-efficacy;
6. Richer interpersonal relationships because you're relaxed; and
7. Enhanced ability to maintain motivation to diet, stop smoking, or exercise.

When you consider the benefits, there is no doubt that you'd want to incorporate this simple, relaxing, and incredibly helpful self-help technique into your weekly schedule. And remember that studies have shown that mindfulness lowers stress hormone levels, and that's something you really want to work on.

In one mindfulness study, which included patients up to 75 years of age, 65% found improvement in mood, and 31% experienced less stress and improved changes in their ability to cope better with daily life activities. Age, therefore, is no roadblock to using and experiencing relief utilizing mindfulness. Some of the participants, interestingly, had described that they had experienced chronic pain for 48 years before coming to the mindfulness training. Pain reduction in the participants was self-reported at 50% overall. So the benefits are unquestionably in your favor and the effort you expend is worth it. You can show yourself that you have more control over things than you thought, so start seeking out resources in the areas we've mentioned here.

Basically, all that is involved is that you place yourself in a quiet environment in your home for a half-hour and present yourself with a calming scene while you allow yourself to just remain "in the moment." I would recommend, however, that if you can find a group that you might join it would be the better choice. It helps to have an instructor who can provide helpful direction and encouragement in the meditation, which you may not always do yourself. Having someplace to go in any wellness plan focuses your attention for the week, provides outlets outside the home and, in so doing, helps in mood enhancement. It's a depression fighter, too, if it's getting you out of your home on a weekly basis.

Again, look at MS programs in your area that are specifically geared to providing meditation programs for members. This step begins, as I said before, the journey of hope and repair for you.

Further Reading

Bennett MP, Zeller JM, Rosenberg L, McCann J. The effect of mirthful laughter on stress and natural killer cell activity. *Altern Ther Health Med*. 2003; 9(2):38–45.

Bennett MP, Lengacher C. Humor and laughter may influence health: III. Laughter and health outcomes. *Evid Based Complement Alternat Med*. 2008;5:37–40

Berk LS, Felten DL, Tan SA, Bittman BB, Westengard J. Modulation of neuroimmune parameters during the eustress of humor-associated mirthful laughter. *Altern Ther Health Med*. 2001;7(2):62–72, 74–76.

Better Health Channel. *Breathing to reduce stress*. Victoria Government, Australia. http://www.betterhealth.vic.gov.au/bhcv2/bhcarticles.nsf/pages/Breathing_to_reduce_stress. Accessed December 2009.

Brown TR, Kraft GH. Exercise and rehabilitation for individuals with multiple sclerosis. *Phys Med Rehabil Clin N Am*. 2005;16(2):513–555.

Burckhardt CS, Anderson KL, Archenholtz B, Hagg O. The Flanagan Quality of Life Scale: evidence of construct validity. *Health Qual Life Outcomes.* 2003;1:59. Available at: http://www.hqlo.com/content/1/1/59. Accessed March 2010.

Cassileth B, Heitzer M, Gubili J. Integrative oncology: Complementary therapies in cancer care. *Cancer Chemother Rev.* 2002;3(4):204–211.

Castellano V, White LJ. Serum brain-derived neurotrophic factor response to aerobic exercise in multiple sclerosis. *J Neurol Sci.* 2008;269: 85–91.

Davidson R, Kabat-Zinn J, Schumacher J, et al. (2003). Alterations in brain and immune function produced by mindfulness meditation. *Psychosom Med.* 2003;65(4):564–570.

Farrell P. (2003). *How to Be Your Own Therapist.* New York: McGraw-Hill.

Fishman LM, Small E. (2007). *Yoga and Multiple Sclerosis: A Journey to Health and Healing.* New York: Demos Medical Publishing.

Haley J. (1993). Uncommon Therapy: The psychiatric techniques of Milton H. Erickson. New York: W. W. Norton & Co.

Harmon M. Exercise as part of everyday life: Staying well. National Multiple Sclerosis Society. 2009.

Hertzog C, Kramer AF, Wilson RS, Lindenberger U. Fit body, fit mind? *Scientific American Mind,* 2009;32–39. Accessed April 2010.

Ludwig DS, Kabat-Zinn J. (2008). Mindfulness in medicine. *J Am Med Association.* 2008;300(11):1350–1352.

Malcomson KS, Dunwoody L, Lowe-Strong AS. Psychosocial interventions in people with multiple sclerosis: a review. *J Neurol.* 2007;254:1–13.

Medical News Today. Exercise helps protect brain of multiple sclerosis patients. Available at: http://www.medicalnewstoday.com/articles/179659.php. Accessed February 2010.

Ostermann T, Schmid W. Music therapy in the treatment of multiple sclerosis: a comprehensive literature review. *Expert Rev Neurother.* 2006;6(4): 469–477.

Page SA, Verhoef MJ, Stebbins RA, Metz LM, Levy JC. The use of complementary and alternative therapies by people with multiple sclerosis. *Chronic Dis Can.* 2003;24(2–3):75–79.

Paulsen P, French R, Sherrill C. (1990). Comparison of wheelchair athletes and nonathletes on selected mood states. *Percept Mot Skills.* 1990;71(3 Pt. 2): 1160–1162.

Prakash RS, Snook EM, Motl RW, Kramer AF. Aerobic fitness is associated with gray matter volume and white matter integrity in multiple sclerosis. *Brain Res.* 2009;1341:41–51. Available at: www.elsevier.com/locate/brainres. Accessed February 2010.

Reynolds G. How much exercise to avoid feeling gloomy? *The New York Times*. 2009. Available at: http://nyti.ms/a0xp4M. Accessed 30, 2009.

Rotter JB. (1966). Generalized expectancies for internal versus external control of reinforcement. *Psychol Monogr.* 1966;80(1):1–28.

Ruscheweyh R, Willemer C, Krüger K, et al. Physical activity and memory functions: an interventional study. *Neurobiol Aging.* Published online September 2009.

Schmid W, Aldridge D. (2004). Active music therapy in the treatment of multiple sclerosis patients: a matched control study. *J Music Ther.* 2004 Fall; 41(3): 225–240.

Seligman MEP. *What You Can Change . . . and What You Can't: The Complete Guide to Successful Self-improvement*. New York: Ballantine Books; 1995.

Seligman MEP. *Authentic Happiness: Using the New Positive Psychology to Realize Your Potential for Lasting Fulfillment*. New York: Free Press; 2002.

Wade L. Wheelchair rugby puts athletes back on the team. *CNN Health*, November 16, 2009. Accessed April 2010.

Wiens ME, Reimer MA, Guyn HL. Music therapy as a treatment method for improving respiratory muscle strength in patients with advanced multiple sclerosis: a pilot study. *Rehabil Nurs.* 1999;24(2):74.

6

Handling Guilt and Maintaining Resilience

Guilt and grief are two of the immediate reactions that can come with a diagnosis of a chronic medical illness. It is a normal reaction to what is perceived as a loss, a sense of the loss of invulnerability regarding our physical health and of seeking an answer to the question, "Why me?" Anyone who has ever had a diagnosis of any chronic medical illness has found him- or herself swimming in a sea of uncertainty. It seems you are alone, unsafe, and vulnerable.

How did this happen? Why did this happen? What did I do that made this happen or what did I fail to do that would have prevented it? Remember how many people interviewed for this book wanted answers to these questions?

Not only does a sense of guilt come into your mind, but you also experience the initial shock of such a diagnosis and, to say the least, it is depressing. However, remember that guilt is one of the components of depression, so this is not unexpected. Depression isn't rational and being an irrational emotion, it piles on the guilt when we are most insecure. We seek answers and one of the immediate places we look is within ourselves and then we begin to extend the circle to everything around us, our work and family history, and our life experiences. This can go on until there is a clarification that, in fact, we are not responsible nor did anyone or anything cause it. It just happened.

It may be in our genetic makeup and that's something over which we had no control. MS does not allow us to decide that if we engage in certain behaviors or fail to do so, we can affect both the diagnosis and the outcome. Although it doesn't allow us to decide about having the diagnosis, it does allow us to work to seek to maintain our level of functioning.

Besides the guilt that we may initially experience, there is guilt in those around us and discomfort that can add to a sense of being a social pariah because of a lack of information or misinformation about MS. Unspoken questions of "Can I catch it?"; "How do I respond to what's just been told to me?"; and "What do I do now?" fill the air. All of these can make you extremely uncomfortable and leave you feeling even somewhat abandoned. However, abandonment is the furthest thing from the minds of those who love you and who are your friends, relatives, coworkers, and passing acquaintances.

Part of the guilt of others may be about the loss they feel and, like you, they may be wondering if they contributed to your diagnosis. Again, it's a natural reaction when you're dealing with an extremely wily and poorly understood disorder. The unknowing makes it that much more uncomfortable for everyone. When we talk about stress, what is the most stressful thing we can think of? It's the unknown, so this is a stressful time for everyone. It is also a time of a realization of some type of loss and, as there is with any loss, a subtle sense of grief or mourning of the loss.

As in any loss or grieving process, this sense of loss and mourning may last for a short time or longer than it might for others. Grief or bereavement isn't something we feel only at the loss of a loved one; it can be experienced when we have lost something of ourselves because of a medical illness. This subject of bereavement and of what was "normal" was researched extensively by Dr. George Bonanno, a professor at Columbia University, in a recent book. He contends that each of us has our own distinct personality and approach to negative information about our loss. How we handle it isn't necessarily according to a set process, but rather something that we determine. When it is our health, a sense of grief does not indicate any lacking in us and should not be seen as abnormal unless it is debilitating to the point that we cannot function for a long time. When this is the case, it calls for a mental health professional to be consulted. Usually, this is a time-limited process that deals with the here and now and the adjustment to a medical illness such as MS.

The question of loss and resilience was also addressed by Dr. Bonanno, who conducted research with female breast cancer survivors. One interesting result of his research was that he found that women who were pleased with their communication and decision-making support with their medical team had more favorable outcomes and a positive outlook on treatment. They found that social support was an important factor in resilience and recovery and that a psychologist can be part of that support system. Therefore, communication and social support from both the professionals and members of your own network will help to allay your fears as they help promote healthy behaviors. The work and the findings with these cancer survivors can be extended, I believe, to those with MS as well.

It is the sense of hope and of personal competency that would appear to be a primary source of initiating psychological changes that bring the mind–body connection into play. When these changes occur, the sense of hope and of action is reinvigorated and the body appears to respond in a positive manner.

Seeking Psychotherapy

Professional help, in terms of psychotherapy, probably isn't going to be what you might have imagined. There is no need to be concerned that a thorough perusal of your childhood experiences with toilet training is on the agenda. If it is, then you've gone to someone who has a totally different orientation than I would choose. I'm a cognitive psychologist, meaning I believe in dealing with the here and now and with offering ways to better adapt to life's challenges.

The choice of a mental health professional, too, is an important one because not everyone is knowledgeable enough about neuropsychiatric medical illnesses or has the training to adequately approach the task. For this reason, I devoted a chapter in my book, *How to Be Your Own Therapist*, to outlining how to find the right professional for you and on interviewing that person to ensure you can work with him or her; yes, interviewing the mental health professional. Would you buy a car without knowing as much as you could about how it performed, what you would be getting for your money, and so forth?

I don't mean to be dismissive, but too many people may be entering therapy without ever asking all the questions they should or without getting direct answers, but instead they were being asked more questions. I don't believe that asking questions when you're buying a service is a sign of mistrust or pathology; some therapists may see it as that and I'd have to wonder why. You are purchasing a service and you have a right to know as much as you need to about how they will provide it, where they were trained, if they have treated a person with MS before, whether they are licensed (and as what), and how their treatment plan will be laid out.

One way you might resolve the problem of finding a qualified psychotherapist is to ask for a referral from one of the MS organizations, a treating neurologist, or someone who has MS or is in therapy who is pleased with the therapeutic relationship. Then, you can arrange for a consultation and see if this person would be someone with whom you were comfortable.

No doubt there are troubling psychological/cognitive components of MS. Some people who receive a diagnosis of MS may take it almost in stride because, at the very least, it has provided relief from a prolonged period of medical problems without explanation. In this way, the prior stress that they may have been experiencing will be lifted because of a period of prolonged uncertainty.

For others, there will be no guilt and little thought that this may affect their lives. However, for others, there will be a sense of loss, almost a bereavement period, after the diagnosis.

Psychotherapy can be very helpful and shouldn't be discounted as an indication of existing mental illness. Although MS may interfere with your mood and your ability to cope as you may have in the past, it does not mean you are mentally ill. You aren't, but you do need some help and you should plan to get all the help you need. You wouldn't go into a battle without the right equipment and this is a battle to maintain your physical and mental health. Notice I said "maintain"? This is exactly what you're going to be doing and it's part of any rehabilitation plan when there's a cognitive component to the illness. Think of it as an opportunity to learn, practice, and hone your social and thinking skills.

The Initial Diagnosis

When Dan was first diagnosed, he experienced some of the same feelings that others had related to me. He said,

> My immediate reaction was, "MS, no problem." I only thought that it would be the mobility part and I had no clue at all that this other stuff was going to go with it. The anger was coming out in all different ways, and my whole family as well as I had

to deal with it. One of my children was in tears because he thought I was going to die. So then I sought out help to deal with whatever I needed to deal with through counseling.

The therapist that I saw right away told me that I didn't need to blame myself for feeling guilty about this because it was nothing that you did. I remember looking at her and thinking, "What is she talking about? Why is she telling me this kind of stuff?" I felt that very strange. In hindsight, as I thought about it, I began to understand that people might deal with it differently than I did. I did not have the guilt. What I had was immediate relief by getting a diagnosis and it told me that I wasn't nuts and the things that were going on were real. I wasn't just making them up. It's not just in my head. That gave me satisfaction.

The main point that I want to make here is that you can *give yourself permission* to experience these emotional ups and downs and all the disappointment that may come with the diagnosis, but that does not mean that there is no hope. We've already seen how people with a diagnosis of MS have effectively managed to bring change into their lives, which has benefitted them and provided a new and unforeseen outlet to work toward helping both themselves and others with MS. The secret, if there is a secret here, is to maintain a sense of resilience. How do you do that? Good question, so let's see what is recommended.

The Road to Resilience

The first thing that you do is, as I've said, allow yourself the feelings that will come with the initial diagnosis. Yes, give yourself permission to do this. I know you may never have thought of it in these terms before, so now is the time for another, subtle life change here.

You may feel like you've been hit by a ton of bricks, not like Dan who experienced relief. You may feel overwhelmed and want to just get away and refuse to believe the diagnosis. You may even be so upset that you don't want to do anything and rehab is the last thing on your mind. No one said you had to quietly accept it and no one is saying it's hopeless, although that, too, may be your initial reaction. There's far too much research now that points to much better outcomes for people with MS. Science has made major strides even in the past decade and each advance has improved treatment outcomes and options.

The second thing to do is to begin to look at several goal areas, which have been touched on in prior chapters but which I would like to consolidate here for you. Let's take a look at some of them.

1. **MS and your outlook.** Your outlook is greatly affected by your sense of control and your ability to "know your MS." Yes, the disease can be seen as an "enemy" but I think you might want to see it as something of a new page in your life. You are going to be proactive. You do this by gathering as much information as you can, on your own, and with the help of MS organizations. Your involvement in your medical care is vital because it will promote a sense of competence and that is precisely what you need right now. Knowledge of the disease also helps you to decrease the stress that lack of knowledge brings. Less stress means more benefit for your immune system. Resolve now that you will *not* take a back seat in your treatment.

2. **Rediscover your ability to act on your own behalf.** A sense of dependence is not going to be in your best interest. This does not mean that you cannot look to others to help you. What it does mean is that waiting to be given information is not the wisest course of action.

3. **Sharpen your problem-solving skills.** When a problem arises, provide yourself with an opportunity to explore multiple options. Usually, there is not one solution to a problem, but many. Whatever course of action you will choose in each of these situations is the one that best fits your individual needs. What's right for one person may not be right for you. *Consider and choose for yourself.* It would be wonderful to have simple answers to some of the complex problems you'll face, but that's not always in the cards.

4. **The Pollyanna approach.** This approach may actually be a good one because, as Annie said in the Broadway play, "the sun will come out tomorrow." Of course, you don't totally deny that there is a problem, but you accept that there is hope. Give yourself some distance, in time, from any problem and you will allow yourself a sense of renewed energy

and changed perspective on the task. If afternoons and evenings are not good times for you, try to shift important decisions to times that are good for you in terms of your energy and mood level. People with MS often find the afternoon and evening is when their energy level is lowest. Immediately in the morning, upon arising, is not a good time for many people, even those who don't have MS. So, give yourself some time after you get out of bed and have your breakfast before any important decision making. *No need to rush unless there's a saber-toothed tiger at the door.*

5. **Lifestyle changes and MS.** *Things in the future will be different,* undoubtedly, but that is not something to dwell on now because it will only promote feelings of helplessness and deepen any depression you may be experiencing. Look toward what you can do and how you can make changes that are useful and important to you. Maintaining this positive outlook is something you will continue to work on because your mood will change and that has to be taken into consideration when deciding on change. This is normal. No one maintains a totally positive outlook 24 hours a day, 7 days a week. You can't be expected to do this, either. Some days you're going to be an absolute ogre, but you'll work on that from now on because *you already know this in advance.*

6. **Nothing is written in stone.** Any changes you make and any plans you have should be seen as a *work in progress.* Everyone's life plan, in fact, should be seen in this perspective because it allows for change that is inevitable and wise. You may make some decisions at one point in your life and then, for reasons unforeseen previously, you may now need to revise these plans. When you do, you are acting wisely. Even resolutions you may make may need to be brought into line with new challenges you could find yourself facing in the future.

7. **Don't buy into the myths.** We've seen that advances in research are opening up new areas with great promise in terms of exercise for people with MS. As was detailed by Dr. Gold, there are many, previously unknown benefits to

exercise that include not only mood enhancement and stress and anxiety reduction with potential pain relief, but also likely potential brain enhancement. The latter includes possible brain growth in terms of neural connections. The brain has incredible abilities, which have not yet been realized and growth and rejuvenation may be two of them. *Keep up on the news.* Remember that exercise doesn't have to be entirely physical and can be mental or have a limited physical component as in video and TV-connected game modules. Talk to a rehab counselor about your own in-home plan.

8. **Reach out to others**. *There's no reason you have to reinvent the wheel* because other people have done the work before you. Now what you need to do is to find them and to work with them. When you do, you can't be expected to know everything and that's the reason you're going to them. They are the experts; you are the student who will intelligently question them.

   Good students do not accept and swallow the information that is given to them but consider questions and open dialogues on this information with the expert. If I were to think that it might be good to bring one good thing back from the 70s, it would be "question authority." But don't question just to prove you can be irritating; question because you need to understand things and these questions should be stated in a way that permits you to fully understand.

9. **Maintain a dialogue with yourself.** As you've seen, some people use journaling to do this because they find that putting their thoughts down on paper helps them to both reinforce and revise what they want to do or say. I also recommend "self-talk" as a way of directly communicating in multiple ways with your brain's memory centers. Verbalizing and hearing what you're saying can be quite helpful. Yes, intelligent people do talk to themselves.

10. **Be good to yourself.** Too often we forget that we not only have a right to be treated well, but we also have a need to treat ourselves well. Please remember this statement from an ancient philosopher who said, "If I am not for myself, then who will be for me?" This does not indicate an egotistical,

selfish, or self-involved problem or disorder, but a reasonable understanding of the need to care for one's self. Taking care of yourself is not pathology, it is health promoting. So, *take time out for pleasure and creative nonsense.* Yes, nonsense. Maintaining a deadly serious demeanor and attitude is going to do more harm than good, so "swing for the fences" and enjoy it.

If you would find it useful, copy these 10 items and put the list on the front of your refrigerator, your computer monitor, or wherever you find it would be most useful. Several times during the day, go over these "new rules" for yourself as a refresher when you tend to find you need a little pep talk.

Further Reading

Bonanno GA. *The Other Side of Sadness: What the New Science of Bereavement Tells Us About Life After Loss.* New York, NY: Basic Books; 2009.

Gold SM, Irwin MR. Depression and immunity inflammation and depressive symptoms in multiple sclerosis. *Neurol Clin,* 2006;24(3):507–519.

Gold SM, Mohr DC, Huitinga I, Flachenecker P, et al. (2005) The role of stress-response systems for the pathogenesis and progression of MS. *Trends Immunol,* 2005;26(12):644–652. Available at: http://www.direct-ms.org/pdf/ImmunologyMS/GoldStressMS.pdf. Accessed September 15, 2010.

Kaplin A. Depression in multiple sclerosis. In: Cohen JA, Rudick RA eds. *Multiple Sclerosis Therapeutics.* 3rd ed. London, England: Informa Healthcare; 2007.

Lam WWT, Bonanno GA, Mancini AD, Ho S, et al. Trajectories of psychological distress among Chinese women diagnosed with breast cancer. *Psychooncology* [published online]. December 11, 2009. Available at: http://onlinelibrary.wiley.com/doi/10.1002/pon.1658/abstract. Accessed September 15, 2010.

7

Maximizing Memory to Combat Depression

Memory is the essential part of our minds, which makes each of us a unique individual. It is our essence, our history book, our planner, and the storehouse of our past, present, and future. Since the design of the first intelligence tests in the early 20th century, memory has played an important role in testing multiple abilities and, unfortunately, it has always been seen as a measure of intelligence. This could not be further from the truth because we know that intelligence is much more than memory or memorizing information or any type of material. Television quiz shows have done a great deal to reinforce this idea of memory and intelligence going hand-in-hand and erroneously giving the impression that anyone who has a superior memory for facts is, of course, of superior intelligence. If that were the case, individuals with the disorder known as savant syndrome (i.e., Rain Man syndrome) would be at the top of the IQ scale. However, they don't score in that range and are usually found within the range indicating mental retardation.

In fact, intelligence tests may not be a very good measure of anything and may not tap all the types of "intelligence" that we have. Psychologists often jokingly comment on this as circular—intelligence tests test whatever intelligence tests measure. Work completed within the past several decades by psychologists has indicated that intelligence is much broader and, in fact, even memory is broader than the common understanding of it.

When we think or talk about memory, it is primarily the type of memory that depends on our cognition, in other words, our thoughts. Memory itself actually includes all of the senses. Therefore, we have memory for touch, smell, taste, sound, vision, and our working memory, which is actively involved in our thinking processes. Unknowingly, we use all of this memory-processing power, but much of what we do in terms of trying to strengthen our memory is directed to only the thinking portion of memory. Rehabilitation experts may disagree with me on this, but in my review of the literature, there doesn't seem to be enough in the way of a multisensorial approach to memory.

Because it is still felt that memory is solidly linked to intelligence, when anyone begins to experience a decline or decrease in their memory skills, it is extremely upsetting because they may begin to equate it with a form of dementia. Multiple sclerosis (MS), which has an effect on cognitive functioning, can make people feel as if they are "slipping" as well. Yes, it can affect memory, but individuals with MS can benefit from various memory enhancement techniques as well as techniques they have devised on their own. There are memory prompts that people have come up with on their own and they work very well for them. No one needs to be a memory researcher to do this.

Memory isn't a simple matter of trying to use techniques to remember facts, names, schedules, and so on. It is an index of how well we may be functioning with regard to several other things, such as *depression*, *anxiety*, and *sleep*, which play pivotal roles in memory. MS can bring with it experiences of decreased memory and concentration, which leads to intensifying existing anxiety and depression, and this can affect self-esteem. Thus, the cycle begins, which leads to more negative feedback and a yet greater lowering of self-esteem and feelings of incompetence.

There is, therefore, no one item that stands alone because anxiety, depression, and self-esteem are intimately linked. Combating any memory problem will have a positive effect on combating changes in mood and levels of anxiety. It goes without saying that MS may cause some brain impairment; however, there are many memory pathways in the brain that can benefit from training. Some of these pathways may not yet be known and it's my contention that the brain is "the final frontier," not outer space.

The Five Factors Involved in Memory

A survey of some of the things that can affect the sharpness of anyone's memory, even in the absence of MS, points to five contributory factors. These five factors all work together and are involved in memory in some way, whether or not you have MS. They include:

1. Depression
2. Anxiety
3. Pain
4. Sleep
5. Medication

How are the five related? Let's take a look at two of them and tease out the complexity involved in memory.

Depression brings with it an inability to sleep or to maintain restorative sleep, or results in early morning arising. Early morning arising, say at 4 AM or so, is most characteristic of major depression and is used as a diagnostic indicator. It robs us of the sleep that is essential for our bodies to adequately function and, also, for mood regulation.

Prolonged major depression has been shown to result in damage to vital areas of the brain that contribute to memory maintenance (e.g., the hippocampus), in particular. The hippocampus is one of the primary centers of memory preservation and acquisition, so anything we can do to improve its functioning, such as addressing ways to decrease depression, is imperative.

Sleep, along with depression, plays a major role because depression interferes with sleep and sleep disruption has a negative effect on memory and concentration during the day. As it is, sleep appears to be given inadequate attention in most people's lives and we often hear them remarking about how little sleep they actually "need." The sleep research contradicts this statement with regard to need.

If we are depressed or we are in pain and we do succeed in sleeping, it is fitful with many awakenings during the night. Sleep researchers at Stanford University have, for the past several decades, studied the results of inadequate sleep and believe that this begins an accumulation of a "sleep debt" that has consequences for our daily activities.

In addition to this sleep research, the National Sleep Foundation conducted its own poll in 2008 of health care providers and queried them about the *most common patient complaints related to insomnia or poor sleep quality.* They found the following sleep-related problems:

- Mood changes, 73%
- Attention/concentration problems, 63%
- Problems in family relationships, 42%
- Problematic job performance, 36%

Sleep also appears to be a mediator in our immune system. Dr. Charles Czeisler, chief of sleep medicine at Brigham and Women's Hospital in Boston, in reviewing a study of persons who had less than 7 hours of sleep per night, indicated that they were 5.5 times more likely to come down with a cold than people who slept soundly through the night. This was a huge effect, according to Dr. Czeisler. He stated this indicates that sleep not only affects alertness and perform- ance but has a *major effect on our physical health.*

In another sleep study, conducted by Sheldon Cohen at Carnegie Mellon University, even those who slept 8 hours but had brief interrup- tions in their sleep were 4 times more likely to develop cold symptoms than people who slept 99% to 100% of the time while in bed.

These sleep effects also appeared to carry over into inhibition of the development of antibodies after flu vaccinations. Sleep-deprived subjects developed only half the antibodies that persons who had adequate sleep managed to produce. Dr. Cohen proposed that the underlying mechanism appeared to be related to the release of inflammatory chemicals and an inflammatory process. Sleep, therefore, would appear to share a relationship with the MS process in terms of immune system dysfunction or dysregulation and inflammation.

Sleep researchers refer to normal sleep patterns, the brain waves generated during sleep, as *sleep architecture.* In sleep disruption, these stages of normal sleep are transformed and this results in getting less of the restorative sleep level that is needed. Less restorative sleep in individuals who are already depressed can result in more depression, irritability, and anxiety in a cyclical loop that reinforces the preexisting depression and exacerbates the sleep disruption. This spiraling effect must be short-circuited if we wish to restore restful sleep and positive daytime mood changes.

Sleep Hygiene

Like what has been stated, depression can also have a major impact on our ability to sleep and to get sufficient and uninterrupted sleep. The sleep graph that is charted during a sleep study shows what is called *sleep architecture*, meaning it outlines your stages of sleep during the night. Some stages are necessary for restorative sleep. The charting can assist in clinical determinations regarding the quality of your sleep such as *sleep apnea*, a not-uncommon cause of daytime drowsiness, and possible depression. The relationship between sleep and depression is understandable if you consider that you may be waking up at least 500 times a night because of undiagnosed apnea wherein you are, unknown to you, gasping for breath.

The sleep equation, in fact, works both ways; inadequate sleep can cause depression and fatigue, and depression can lead to inadequate sleep. We now know that sleep does play a role in memory consolidation and the development of depression, which can also affect memory and the integrity of brain structures. The sleep medicine experts provide the following recommendations regarding good sleep habits, or "sleep hygiene":

- Maintain a regular sleep–wake schedule.

- Upon arising, get into bright light (it doesn't have to be sunlight).

- Have some form of exercise during the day, but not prior to sleep at night.

- If possible, avoid afternoon naps. Patients with MS may find this difficult because of afternoon fatigue.

- Limit your intake of caffeine and alcohol. Remember that caffeine is contained in many products and not confined to only coffee or tea.

- Researchers also recommend that you confine your bedroom, as much as possible, to sleep-related activities, so try not to eat, read, or watch TV in bed.

- Your bedroom should have window coverings to exclude as much light as possible during your sleep time.

- For other recommendations, check the Internet for "sleep hygiene" where well-known researchers provide updated information on current sleep discoveries.

Additional research that looked into the question of what is called "wakeful resting" and memory suggests that there are forms of rest that don't involve sleep, but are vital to memory. It revolves around the idea that memory consolidation can take place during our wide-awake times, if we allow it. How do we allow it to set these new memories more firmly into our brain banks? We take time out and rest after any memory tasks. During this coffee break or downtime, the brain is still actively working to help keep those memories for long-term use. So, work at remembering things, but give yourself a bit of a break immediately afterward, and these researchers say there will be improvement.

Anxiety, Pain, Sleep, and Medication

Anxiety is directly related to our pain threshold and we know that MS can bring pain. Pain, therefore, is something beneficial to control or decrease, and any decrease in anxiety can contribute toward this goal. Again, there's a direct relationship to pain, which translates into deepening depression and disruption of sleep. The cycle is continuous and unforgiving unless we become proactive and work against it.

Pain is one of the most mentioned problems that patients with any chronic illness indicate as their primary reason for not being able to sleep. Decreasing anxiety, as was just mentioned, can result in decreased pain and improved sleep.

Sleep not only allows us to allocate time for our bodies to recuperate from the day and to engage in any reparative activities, but it is also a time for consolidating memory and, therefore, vital to memory maintenance or improvement. You just saw how it is affected by depression, anxiety, and pain.

A review of the research indicates that *greater numbers of patients with MS* often have *unrecognized sleep disorders* in excess of the general population. The specific disorders include disordered breathing, insomnia, poor rapid eye movement (REM) sleep, narcolepsy, and restless legs syndrome. All of these may be related to dysfunction of the immune system and the action of inflammatory cytokines.

Medication for many medical or psychological problems can have an effect on both concentration and memory, sleep, or the quality of sleep. Some medications can result in bizarre dreams, which can be quite disturbing and sleep disruptive. It may even be a matter of when you take your medications: morning or night. All of this should be discussed with your physicians.

If you'd like to check on whether or not some of your medications may be involved in this decreased sharpness or disruption of sleep, you can do an Internet search or go to the local library's reference section for the "bible" of pharmaceutical prescribing. This book, the *Physicians' Desk Reference* (PDR), contains information on the medications, the usual dosages, and any side effects listed by the percentage of individuals who indicated each side effect. There are also similar books for over-the-counter (OTC) medications and herbal medicines.

It is not unusual for MS patients to indicate that they have noticed upsetting changes in their memory. Research has indicated that memory impairment is among the most common deficits mentioned by patients with MS to their physicians. These changes may have been brought on by the MS disease process, depression, sleep deprivation, increased anxiety, and may also, in part, be a side effect of medications patients are currently receiving. All of these factors must be considered when evaluating memory impairment because each of them will require a specific intervention.

The interventions may be either of a professional or of a self-help nature, and it is the latter that provides reason for optimism because it means the person can exercise some control him/herself. This bolsters the ever-useful sense of optimism that can provide a potential boost to the immune system of a patient with MS, in addition to any medical interventions.

An interesting study of physical activity and its relationship to memory found that physical activity does have a beneficial effect on cognition regardless of the intensity of the activity. It would, therefore, further bolster the argument for any type of physical activity being useful for body conditioning, balance, sleep, and memory improvement or maintenance. Some studies have indicated that, with advanced age, exercise can provide a means of preventing or delaying the onset of mild cognitive impairment in persons without MS.

One research psychologist, Dr. Ruchika Prakash of Ohio State University, found herself the sudden object of media attention when she and her colleagues announced the results of their work with exercise and cognition in people with MS. It was clearly unexpected but served as an indication of just how much both the public and the media were interested in this story.

"We were contacted by people with MS who were happy that we were doing this research because their doctors had always told them that they had to be careful about exercising." These individuals told her and her team that they believed in exercising and they've been doing a lot of it, and they had seen significant improvement. One person "who wasn't able to walk for a while and started doing exercise is running a marathon." He was an exception, she advised.

> My research is looking at how exercise might improve cognitive functioning. Up until recently, it wasn't considered to show beneficial effects for individuals with MS and there was also, for the longest time, the belief that MS patients experienced very little decline in cognitive functioning. But there's been a dramatic change from that. We now know that cognitive symptoms are found to be the defining feature, so about 65–85% of the population experiences some kind of cognitive deficit.

The initial research started out looking at older adults and exercise, and gradually evolved into looking at people living with MS. "We were doing our research with older adults and realized that a lot of the underlying mechanisms that exercise helps with has to do with increases in the production of nerve growth factor and a lot of research with animals found that it shows an improvement in cognitive functioning."

As Dr. Prakash explained,

> An area of significant deficiencies you see in MS patients are in these nerve growth factors that decline especially when you look at relapse when people go through phases of relapses when their symptoms exacerbate. So we wanted to see if there would be an association between fitness and cognitive improvement in functioning within this population.

Working from this idea that there might be an as-yet-understudied area in nerve growth factor, Dr. Prakash began her research.

> That's how we got started with the research and we've been finding some extremely strong results, which is contrary to the

thinking that exercise was thought to be actually harmful for multiple sclerosis. We've been finding that there is a very strong association between their cognitive functioning on standardized tests where MS patients had always performed extremely poorly.

The area where the most exciting results have been seen is in

processing speed improvements and that applies to very simple cognitive skills that help you to take in information, process it and respond to it. Reaction time is one of the significant deficits where these patients can't process information at a faster rate. What we found was that patients with higher levels of fitness did much better on these tests than non-fit MS patients. In addition to that we put them in MRI scanners and collected both structural data and functional MRI and found improvements in both of those.

The magnetic resonance imaging (MRI) scanned areas Dr. Prakash and her colleagues noted were as follows:

higher fit MS patients had less lesion volume in their brains. From a functional perspective, we gave them a task to do while they were inside the scanner. This task actually measured processing speed. The tasks we used are the most widely used ones by psychologists, neurologists and physicians. Again, there was an important difference between those who were fit as opposed to those who were not fit.

So, the physical evidence and the test-related psychological evidence appeared to point to a positive relationship between exercise and cognitive improvement.

Now, the research is going to be extended. "A new piece of research we hope to do is to compare two groups; one stretching and toning, the other an aerobic exercise group and see if exercise reduces these cognitive deficits." Cause and effect isn't something Dr. Prakash is willing to speculate on because there hasn't been a clinical trial looking at this particular aspect of cognitive functioning. From a future perspective, the result looks very interesting. The research will also look at multiple factors such as gender, disease duration, age, and education, among other variables.

Being a prudent and careful researcher, Dr. Prakash indicated:

At this point, this isn't a clinical intervention because we haven't proven yet that exercise does, in fact, improve cognitive functioning. We only have an association in relapsing and remitting MS so until we actually do the exercise intervention, I'm hesitant to say that exercise, in fact, will reduce cognitive impairment. But there is an association and it is a strong one.

One of my recommendations to the patients that I see at my clinic and to anyone who has contacted me is that we have found this association and if you think it works for you, then you should go ahead and do it, but always be cognizant of your own limitations. That's something to always keep in mind and, if things are not working out, then it's okay to stop.

The question of exercise and raising the core body temperature was also a consideration.

When I first began working in MS research, we knew that MS patients were thermosensitive and that exercise is known to increase body temperature and as a result symptoms could be exacerbated. But if you think from a long-term perspective, even in younger and older adults, if you've been sedentary for awhile and you start exercising, it causes a significant amount of discomfort. That does not mean, necessarily, that it would exacerbate your symptoms.

You might feel uncomfortable and you might not like how your body feels at that time and you'll be sore. But after that, as you start doing it at a much more regular pace, then you start seeing improvement. One of the things that we also want to do is to see how aquatic therapy helps.

We're doing a study right now in which participants run quite a bit. We collect how much they exercise, how much they are walking, etc. We have this one participant who had been in a wheelchair and who biked about 43 miles in one day and he does about 33 miles on alternate days. He was an athlete before he got MS.

This was an extraordinary result, Dr. Prakash cautioned, and not the usual improvement that might be expected. There have also been patients with MS at the clinic who initiated their own exercise programs.

"I know of someone who was just about in a wheelchair. He got a physical trainer and he started exercising slowly and has been walking just fine. He exercises about 45 minutes every day and he is very active in his profession." Previously, it had been assumed that he would have to leave his position because of his increasing disability.

The association between mood states and exercise is also of interest to Dr. Prakash.

> Right now, we're also studying the association between cognitive functioning and depression and how that's affected by exercise. We're looking to see if people who exercise more are less depressed and as a result have better cognitive functioning as opposed to people who don't exercise that much and are more depressed and have worse cognitive functioning. You can definitely see the connection in improving their quality of life and, similarly, affecting how they interact socially and how this would influence every aspect of their lives.

It is Dr. Prakash's belief that depression in MS is a topic that is understudied. Patients come to her facility and they score significantly high on depression measures. Her team is starting an MS clinic to deal with cognitive functioning and depression in MS. One of the things she will be doing is neuropsychological evaluations and, in addition, individualized cognitive therapy for patients with MS. The idea is to see if cognitive behavioral therapy will also reduce depression within this population. Then they will go another step further to look at combining cognitive therapy with both exercise and medication-based therapy.

Their aim is to address as many aspects of MS as they can and to include in their treatment regimes all the therapies that have been found in any way to be beneficial (e.g., exercise, psychotherapy, and medication for depression, if needed).

Everyday Memory Problems

One of the people interviewed for this book, Anna, had noticed some word-finding difficulty; the medical term for this is *aphasia*.

> There are times when I'm speaking and I have problems, or delays, in trying to find what I want to say. Eventually, however,

it will come to me, but it's like a delayed reaction. But I keep pushing myself until it comes to me and eventually it does come back.

Sometimes I'll go into a room and I'll forget what I went in for, and it will get me a little upset. I keep pushing myself and try to remember what it was. I even do word association as a way to deal with this until it pops back into my mind. Around the house, I keep lists so I can remember what I need to do.

Memory specialists would suggest the use of self-repetition here: repeating what you are going to get in the kitchen until you get hold of that item in your hand or begin to work on the project you had in mind. This process, also called *rehearsal*, keeps the thought in short-term memory, where it belongs, because you won't need it for more than the next few minutes.

A man who had been involved in demanding, professional work indicated that:

I started to experience memory problems as far as being able to recall. I had a job that required that I have a sharp mind at the time. My train of thought was being derailed constantly and I wasn't able to put it back on the track.

Sometimes, I needed to have facts at my fingertips and there was no reason that my train of thought should have been derailed at all. It was obvious to me that I was struggling to recall basic facts and information about projects that I was working on. I couldn't mentally dance fast enough to get by. Fortunately, it was a short period of time for me to understand what was going on and I made the decision that I had to retire.

He was in a profession in which clients relied on his ability to be fast and precise with his information and recommendations, and his sense of duty to them weighed heavily on his mind.

No client experienced any damage, nor was anything detrimental done to any of them, but it took me some time to prepare for my work and much longer to accomplish the same thing. This was something that, previously, I might be able to do in an hour or an hour and a half. Now, maybe it took a full weekend for me to prepare and even then I wasn't good to go and hit the ground running. On Monday morning, I would still have to refresh the information that I had jammed into my brain and which wasn't on the tip of my tongue, where it normally would be.

A few visits to one neurologist resulted in little help with his problems, but change was about to happen.

The first neurologist I saw did the best thing for me that she could have done and that was to refer me to someone else. This second neurologist brought in a neuropsychologist, because the first neurologist's advice, that I relax and take it easy and take some time off, isn't normally a method of treatment for MS. MS isn't resolved by relaxing.

The [second] neuropsychologist ran me through a day or two of a battery of tests that I didn't understand, and the neuropsychologist ended up bringing in a different neurologist who was much more acquainted with my difficulty and had a deeper understanding of the treatments that would be required.

That's the first time I heard cognitive or mental activity associated with MS and the brain. All of the brochures and all of the information that I had been presented with had nothing with the mind. It was all physical. I had read about numbness and loss of equilibrium and optic neuritis and that various parts of my body would shut down because of this disorder but there was nothing dealing with your mind. This neuropsychologist and neurologist got it. They understood from the moment I walked in the door.

When the diagnosis was made, it was actually a relief; something many people with MS experience.

The doctors showed me the results of the tests, which was the best and worst thing to show me because they relieved my mind that this was not Alzheimer's, this wasn't Parkinson's, and it wasn't anything else. Whatever my intelligence level was it was still there, somewhere, and they said that the problem was access. It's just like with your leg; the muscles are still there, but your ability to have it function in the same capacity as it used to function is compromised.

I realized it was the same thing with my cognitive, my thinking function. My memories were all still there, they just kind of shifted around and I couldn't rely on them when I needed them. But I shouldn't freak out and I should just know that it would pass.

These memory problems are something that he must address on a daily basis.

My memory has changed regarding the length of time that I need to grasp a thought. It's not like what started with a 15-second delay is now taking significantly more time for me. It's more the frequency with which it happens.

A day doesn't go by where I don't get lost. I'll be driving, almost on any given day, and I have to constantly remind myself with notes in the car. The notes tell me why I'm going there and where I'm going because I may not remember why I got into the car in the first place.

So the frequency of that continues, and it continues to increase but the duration of each does not seem to extend. And this will expand into different people, different locations, different items, and it's not as though I had my mind on any one thing.

The very things that he was mentioning as being problematic were the subject of research. One study of memory in patients with MS indicated that the *most frequently forgotten things* were names and faces of individuals they knew, locations of frequently used objects such as their keys, eyeglasses, and so forth, and appointments and the date on which the appointments were to occur.

10 Tips for Improving Memory

Memory, as you've just seen, is a combination of things from our level of anxiety, our mood, our pain level, and even how well we sleep each night. But there are tips that have been found helpful and are used by many people. Here are some of the things that both health professionals and patients use:

1. *Organize* in terms of designating a specific spot in your home, your car, or your office for things like your mail,

your bills, and your keys. This spot should also have a pad or notebook/calendar with pens so that you can quickly jot down things you need to remember. Make this, as they say in TV production studios, "home base" where everything happens and where you can get whatever information you need.

In other words, you need a set routine and you need to stick to it. Routines help lessen anxiety and are going to prove invaluable here. Whatever way you organize, keep faithful to the KISS (keep it simple, stupid) imperative that all graduate students are taught when they begin working on their dissertations. Simple is best and the fewer steps to recall to do something, the better.

2. *Utilize* a day planner, cell phone with calendar, or whatever you prefer when you leave your home, *whenever* you leave your home. A quick trip to the grocery store is included here because you may need to note something in your planner while you're out. Scraps of paper won't do the job, so putting the reminder on one of them means you've got a problem in the making.

If you're so inclined, use a personal digital assistant (PDA) like a BlackBerry or some other phone/appointment device. These, however, need to be backed up to your computer because their memories can sometimes get mixed up as well, so don't depend on them solely. Small digital voice recorders are now inexpensive enough that you can leave notes to yourself on them and then plug the recorder into your computer at home for retrieval. Keep in mind the watchword of realtors (with a little modification here): *back up, back up, back up.*

3. *Computerize* with pop-up reminders. There are programs that can keep your calendar and also put a daily "to do" list for you on your screen as you boot up your computer each day. Pop-up reminders can be scheduled to flag important dates, times, or anything you have scheduled. Not everything has to be expensive, because there are freeware programs on safe Internet sites. We've added a few of these sites in our Resources section of this book.

4. *"Simplify"* (i.e., be creative) and break everything down into smaller tasks so they don't become overwhelming. The turtle, not the hare, wins the race, remember? And take a break if you suddenly feel something is just too much to handle. You're entitled to your own "coffee breaks" in your life and you can just use a bit of relaxation breathing or imagery to help get things sorted out again.

5. *Asking* for help is *always* allowed. In fact, it's highly recommended. You don't have to know all the answers, so give yourself a break and ask someone else to help you anywhere you need help. One woman said she couldn't remember which was the front and which was the back of a T-shirt. Another woman said that even remembering her name, when she's stressed, can be a problem.

   Anxiety can cause memory problems in anyone, even someone without MS. I know of a woman who went to the local licensing office to get her driver's license. After a written exam, she had to read an eye chart on the wall. "I looked at the chart and I could see it, but I couldn't remember the alphabet. I was that anxious about getting my license that, for a few moments, I forgot the alphabet." It can be just that simple and understandably upsetting, and it may mean you start out feeling too embarrassed to ask someone for help. But, it's not you; it's the illness and everyone will understand. If they don't, they need to be educated about the illness. Refer them, gently, to the MS Web site: www.nationalmssociety.org.

6. *Finding your way home*, or to any other place for that matter, doesn't need to be anxiety evoking because we now have global positioning system (GPS) devices that go in our cars. You can program it for several destinations (your home is one of them, maybe the post office, your office, the market, etc.) and it will give you *voice commands* for every turn and tell you, *in advance*, when you are coming to an exit or turn.

   If you prefer a more visual approach, you can make maps with your computer and boldly outline the route.

Break the route down into simple steps; then, print step-by-step instructions below each portion of the route. Of course, this should be used as a refresher, not something you keep looking at while you're driving. Put them in a folder and keep them next to the driver's seat.

Visual diagrams are often easier to remember than word descriptions, so these maps may be much better than just written instructions to anyplace. Use color markers to indicate stop signs, traffic signals, and turns you have to make. In fact, drawing, by hand, is one of the methods used in college biology classes to teach complex structures seen under a microscope. *Drawing it reinforces it and aids memory.*

7. *Sign up for MyBrainGames* (www.MyMSMyWay.com), a collaborative effort of business and the National MS Society. Here you will find not only information on assistive technology (AT) such as voice recognition software and "talking" computer capability but also cognition-enhancing games to serve as memory aids. The game has three parts—shopping list, word connect, and round-up—and each one will keep track of your score and help you stay on track with your practice.

Repetition and practice are key to any memory aids you may use, so this one fits in nicely and is visual with on-screen aids to change font size, contrast, and other variables. Remember the many types of sense memories I mentioned earlier? Here is where you use several of them: touch, vision, possibly sound, and cognitive processing. When I say cognitive processing, of course, I'm talking about the thinking/planning portion of memory.

One extra tip about reading and memory—read everything three times. All college students are told that that's the best way to remember anything you've read, as well as making notes in the margin of your books. On your personal computer screen, you can place "sticky notes" or use highlighting built into the computer program you're using.

8. *Mnemonics* is a way of coming up with a clever rhyme or play on words that will help you remember something. The more nonsensical the rhyme, the easier it can be to use as a memory aid. I remember taking a geology class in college and the professor wanted us to remember something about minerals cooling from volcanoes. We students knew nothing about lava or volcanoes, but he soon helped us with a sentence that included something like "All older ants love baby ants" and another for the geologic periods that went something like "Put ears on my plate please Hortense," or "Please eliminate old men playing poker honestly."

   If you are more visual, and we do find that visuals can be especially helpful for many people, make up comical scenes in your mind. Some people use mental "road maps" to remember things and they take a mental trip down a familiar street and put things in stores or on shelves.

   This road map method is similar to an elaborate memory technique used by a man who actually *couldn't forget*. His name was "S" and he was tested for several decades by the famous Russian neuropsychologist A.R. Luria. No matter when he was tested, S had perfect recall and used everything from letters, colors, and objects in his elaborate memory schemes.

9. *Link and story method.* There's also something called the "link and story" method, which is very similar to the technique used by S, in which a story was constructed using items that needed to be remembered. Another method uses rhyming a number with a word that rhymes with it and then making a sentence from that. Here's one that illustrates this point:

   Example: To remember 5,479, you might come up with: A hive (5) pours (4) heavenly (7) pine (9). Silly? Yes, but that's what it's supposed to be so that you will remember it.

   We've given you a link to an Internet site for this and several other memory methods in our Resources section.

One of the resources to which we've pointed has an entire listing of how to remember just numbers, which is:

Number	Rhymes With
1	bun
2	shoe
3	tree
4	pour or paw
5	hive
6	bricks
7	heaven
8	gate
9	pine
10	hen

As a starter, this is a pretty good one and one with which you can begin practicing right away. But you can also find words that you'd prefer and make a list of those and keep it somewhere near home base.

You get the point; it has to be ridiculous and, maybe, just a bit comical to make you laugh as you use it. You make up your own rhymes and when you do, you are using "self-generated encoding," which means you are using your own memory schemes that you've created. We'll discuss self-generated memories in the next section.

10. *Music as a mnemonic device.* Music can serve as a memory cue, as noted in research on music therapy. Because we know that information, once stored in long-term memory, must be retrieved via some technique that will be easy to learn and simple to use and will involve minimal effort, music has been seen as something that can meet all of these requirements. Music provides a means to organize material and this may be the reason we recall that simple song from our childhood where we learned our ABCs. Remember it? Familiar melodies work best, and if you can put anything into a song that you've remembered, or one you construct yourself, it can be very helpful.

It should be repetitive and simple, as the researchers indicate, such as a folk or children's song. This method has proved to be highly successful with learning scientific information, telephone numbers, and even the names of professional sports players. Once information is processed with musical cues, it appears that it is much easier to both retrieve and relearn after a period of disuse. The key to success was actively rehearsing and practicing over a period of time. We only need to consider those radio and TV commercial jingles we heard many years ago that stuck with us to understand the true power of music and memory. How many can you recall right now?

Self-Generated Memories

The topic of self-generated learning is one that is being researched by Dr. Nancy Chiaravalloti, a clinical neuropsychologist and research director of the Kessler Research Center in New Jersey. Dr. Chiaravalloti noted that:

> In MS, we wanted to see if self-generated memory held up and then if you could apply it to everyday life.
>
> We tried to get something novel that patients could use and that their significant others could use. We found, when we tested self-generated memory in laboratory studies, that MS patients perform at levels that are equivalent to healthy individuals' performance under normal learning conditions. So we were essentially able to raise their levels of learning and memory up to normal levels. It was very clear that there was a benefit to using this technique.
>
> We are now taking self-generation and applying it to daily life. What we found in the first studies that we've run is that, indeed, it does help in everyday tasks like a cooking task as well as managing financial tasks.

These tips on memory enhancement are wonderful. But don't give up the methods you have come up with on your own. As Dr. Chiaravalloti added, "The first thing I would tell anyone is that it's very important for them to continue engaging in cognitive challenging tasks such as crossword puzzles, word searches, and reading newspapers." Even though the tasks might be getting difficult, it's important to continue engaging in the task.

Once you establish that prior efforts also play a role, then the newer techniques are explored. Dr. Chiaravalloti said,

> The next thing I would tell them is that there are novel techniques out there that would help them with their everyday memory. We're still in the early stages, but things like generating your own information would help you to remember things in your daily life.
>
> Instead of somebody giving you a shopping list when you have to go to the store, if you know that you're going to have problems remembering your list of items when you go into the store, it's better if you generate that list yourself than to have your spouse generate it for you. You may not remember them saying, "Pick up these items." If you try to use that mental list of things, chances are you may very well have a problem remembering the items.

Examples, based on this current perspective of memory, include:

- Taking a *look at the refrigerator yourself*, if you are going grocery shopping;
- *Determining what items you need*; and
- *Writing the items down yourself*. This reinforces memory in that you first *make a decision* on what is needed, *use that information* in short-term memory, and then *make a written list*. The effort put in making that list yourself is also an aid in memory.

All of these steps support your likelihood of remembering the list. As memory research becomes advanced, there is no reason to not incorporate everything you've devised on your own and that has worked for you. Research, in fact, often depends on making advances by taking advantage of things already discovered by patients and then designing experiments around these patient-generated behaviors. One of your individual memory-boosting techniques just might be an important breakthrough researchers are looking for.

Avoid Repetition as a Memory Aid

One thing that Dr. Chiaravalloti says should be avoided, surprisingly, is repetition. But what she is referring to is not what I mentioned about repetition earlier in this chapter. She is referring to how people fail to realize that just telling someone something, time and time again, is not going to get the task done.

> Repetition in and of itself is not helpful. We did a study that looked simply at repetition and we wanted to see whether people who had more repetitions remembered things better than people who received fewer repetitions. In MS, the answer was, "No."
>
> Just repeating the information to someone, essentially, doesn't do any good. If a spouse or someone else just keeps saying the same thing over and over in the same manner, it won't help. The problem here, and which is important, is that the spouses get extremely frustrated when their significant other isn't remembering something. So, they repeat things and then they get more frustrated because they keep repeating it and it can have a damaging effect on the relationship. It's really important for families to understand that just repeating things doesn't help. So don't keep using it because it won't work.

An alternative that Dr. Chiaravalloti suggests is:

> Instead of constantly repeating something the same way, try saying something and then asking the person a question about it. In other words, make it a conversation, not an inquisition or an unpleasant exercise in memory difficulties.
>
> What you're doing is giving the person an opportunity to generate their own information and guiding them in terms of what information you're asking them to generate.

In other words, it's what psychologists call a *cueing technique*. Cueing aids retrieval.

How does this work better than repetition, something we've always thought worked best? Dr. Chiaravalloti said:

> There are two ways of thinking about why self-generation works better. One is that you are priming the brain's frontal

executive system to call up those memories. The second is that you are engaging deeper levels of memory in the brain and more links are being created to that memory. It works, so there's no reason not to use it. I actually use it in my daily life.

In addition to this type of question-and-answer technique, she suggested something students have used for quite a long time: self-testing. "Another novel effect that has been important in cognitive psychology and which is now being used here is the 'testing effect.' It's a tip everyone was taught to use in college. If you test yourself on information, you'll remember it better than if it were just given to you." So, it's the same as that self-generated list we just saw in the last few paragraphs. Now, you question yourself and provide that memory tug that you need on your own.

We applied this idea in a project with a group of patients with MS and we had significant results. If a person is tested on information, we found that it holds true with these patients, too. They were better able to remember it than when it was simply provided to them over and over again. Self-testing works, too, and it works very well.

In the study what we did was present people with words and some words were just presented over and over again. Other words were presented with another word paired with it. Then we tested them by giving them only the first word and they had to remember the second (the paired word).

How people can use this to remember something in daily life, according to Dr. Chiaravalloti, is by testing themselves. "You'll be able to remember that information better."

This work comes out of other studies in which the researchers tried to figure out the problem areas of memory. Dr. Chiaravalloti said, "*Acquisition, consolidation and retrieval* is how we break memory down. We found that the problem in MS patients was in acquisition and consolidation, but not retrieval." This statement may come as a surprise to anyone with MS because they've always assumed it was their retrieval of things in memory that was the problem.

"As a result of this, all of our subsequent studies have focused on boosting learning and improving a patient's ability to initially acquire information. We've also used 'dual encoding' such as trying to remember some verbal information and then making a picture of it in the individuals' minds," Dr. Chiaravalloti said.

So, they are using more of those sense memories we mentioned earlier in this book. Remember that all the senses can aid in memory, so the more senses put to the task, the better the outcome would be.

"Spouses, family members and others are in a position to apply self-generation and to begin cueing the MS individual with something that suggests what might be needed." The important point to remember is not to say what you're looking for.

"For example, 'I ran out of that stuff you use for shaving.' The other person has to self-generate the word for the item (shaving cream) in response to this cue. Cueing is repeated until a specific answer is generated by the person with MS." At first, this may seem laborious, but learning any new way of relating to someone can take time, but the effort is not without merit. The one thing to remember is not to give up. Too often, when something doesn't immediately feel comfortable or seem to be producing the result you want, the tendency is to stamp it as "no good" or "doesn't work for me," but time is on your side. Use it wisely.

A Partner's Role

Much of what we've provided on memory in this chapter, as you can see, deals primarily with only the individual who has MS. Although research and rehabilitation have concentrated on developing more sophisticated techniques for memory enhancement, there has been little in the way of sharing these advances with spouses, partners, or others involved with the affected individual. Educating a larger audience for these memory techniques to improve the memory abilities of anyone with MS is one of the primary efforts now.

If a loved one wants to help their partner with memory impairment by using cueing, it would seem reasonable that training sessions, specifically for this purpose, should be set up. There should also be a means to evaluate the effectiveness of this approach. The individual with MS should not be expected to assume this task entirely alone. It is my recommendation, therefore, that memory enhancement be a two-person project. In this way, both the person who needs assistance and the partner can reinforce what each other is learning. Such a cooperative effort could prove more fruitful than one based solely on a single individual's efforts. I would suggest, therefore, that anyone reading this book and the memory tips included in it share the information with a significant person in their life. Begin to tag-team memory enhancement and the result is bound to be more significant.

Remoralization

Failing memory can lead to what Dr. Adam Kaplin, a psychiatrist specializing in the biological basis of depression and cognitive impairment in MS at Johns Hopkins University School of Medicine, referred to as feelings of failure, being overwhelmed, "and the sense of isolation that collectively represent demoralization."

It is Kaplin's contention that this sense of demoralization is at the heart of the memory and daily living problems of people with MS, and he has advised, in his writings, to teach remoralization. Kaplin, in other words, believes in helping patients with MS *learn new problem-solving skills to establish a sense of mastery*, and he suggests ways to accomplish this.

Remoralization, according to Dr. Kaplin, can begin with following these additional tips *for daily living skills*:

- *Building rest periods into an afternoon schedule* to deal with the fatigue that leads to depression and a sense of helplessness
- Establishing *individual or group support* to deal with the sense of isolation
- Education regarding *coping strategies*
- *Shopping at off-peak hours* to minimize the feeling of being rushed, which can contribute to anxiety and increase a sense of hopelessness
- *Reexamining beliefs* about the gains you've made and seeing even the smallest of gains as significant

The whole concept of remoralization is one of making adjustments and adaptations to provide a more reasonable manner in which to do things. The cognitive portion helps you to evaluate what you need/want to do in light of *your abilities*. Placing everything within this new dynamic puts you in a better frame of mind, vis-à-vis your abilities, and *enables you to decrease life stressors*.

There are no hard-and-fast rules for doing any of this because, if there were, then you might be led to a failure experience instead of a positive one. You could come to believe that if you couldn't follow the rules, then you couldn't do anything or, similarly, if you couldn't accomplish the task according to these strict rules, you are worthless.

I know this sounds rather simplistic, and you might even find it a little offensive, but *depression can easily lead you to this type of thinking*. You decide what you, reasonably, can do with the ability and energy you have, and then you plan accordingly.

Maintaining the perspective that things can be seen from many different mental angles also helps when trying to come up with changes in your outlook on yourself and your life. Psychologists call this *cognitive restructuring*, but you can see it as taking a fresh approach to an existing challenge.

Further Reading

Basso MR, Lowery N, Chormley C, Combs D, Johnson J. Self-generated learning in people with multiple sclerosis. *J Int Neuropsychol Soc.* September 2006;12(5):640–648.

Brass SD, Duquette P, Proulx-Therrien J, Auerbach S. Sleep disorders in patients with multiple sclerosis. *Sleep Med Rev.* 2009;7:1–9.

Chiaravalloti N, DeLuca J, Moore N, Ricker JH. Cognitive remediation as treatment for new learning deficits in multiple sclerosis. *Int J MS Care.* 2002; 4:77.

Chiaravalloti N, Demaree H, Gaudino EA, DeLuca J.Can the repetition effect maximize learning in multiple sclerosis? *Clin Rehabil.* February 2003;17 (1):58–68.

Cooney E. Good night's sleep may prevent a cold, study finds. Boston: Boston Globe, Div. of The New York Times Co.; January 13, 2009. Available at: http://www.boston.com/news/nation/articles/2009/01/13/good_nights_sleep _may_prevent_a_cold_study_finds/. Accessed December 20, 2009.

Dement W. Sleepless at Stanford. What all undergraduates should know about how their sleeping lives affect their waking lives. Stanford University Center of Excellence for the Diagnosis and Treatment of Sleep Disorders, Stanford University. September 1997. Available at: http://www.stanford.edu /~dement/sleepless.html. Accessed January 2010.

Kaplin A. Depression in multiple sclerosis. In: Cohen JA, Rudick RA, eds. *Multiple Sclerosis Therapeutics*. 3rd ed. London: Informa Healthcare; 2007: 825–844.

Luria AR. *The mind of a mnemonist: A little book about a vast memory.* Cambridge: Harvard University Press; 1987.

Moore KS, Peterson DA, O'Shea G, McIntosh GC, Thaut MH. The effectiveness of music as a mnemonic device on recognition memory for people with multiple sclerosis. *J Music Ther.* Fall 2008;45(3):307–329.

National Sleep Foundation. Depression and sleep: Sleep survey of healthcare professionals. 2005. Available at: http://www.sleepfoundation.org/article /sleep-topics/depression-and-sleep. Accessed December 19, 2009.

Newland PK, Naismith RT, Ullione, M. The impact of pain and other symptoms on quality of life in women with relapsing-remitting multiple sclerosis. *J Neurosci Nurs.* December 2009;41(6):322–328.

Paddock C. Juggling boosts brain connections. *Medical News Today.* October 12, 2009. Available at: http://www.medicalnewstoday.com/articles/167052.php. Accessed September 15, 2010.

PDR: Physicians' Desk Reference 2010. PDR Network LLC; 2010.

PDR: Guide to Over-the-Counter Drugs. Merck & Co. Available at: http://bit .ly/d7gmQB. Accessed September 15, 2010.

PDR for Herbal Medicines (Physicians' Desk Reference for Herbal Medicines). 1st ed. Montvale, NJ: Thomson Reuters Healthcare.

Ruscheweyh R, Willemer C, Kruger K, Duning T, et al. Physical activity and memory functions: An interventional study. *Neurobiol Aging.* August 2009. Published online September 1, 2009. Available at: http://bit.ly/buFwsL. Accessed September 15, 2010.

Tambini A, Ketz N, Davachi, L. Enhanced brain correlations during rest are related to memory for recent experiences. *Neuron.* January 2010;65(2): 280–290.

Weber B, Kim Peek, Inspiration for 'Rain Man,' Dies at 58. *New York Times.* December 26, 2009. Available at: http://www.nytimes.com/2009/12/27/us /27peek.html. Accessed September 15, 2010.

8

Coping Strategies for Every Day

Stress is a part of everyday life. We find it not only in the things that are unpleasant or problematic in our lives but also in those instances where we feel we should experience nothing but joy. Keeping this thought in mind, you can understand that stress can come from the birth of a child, birthday parties, weddings, job promotions, the purchase of a new home, a windfall in the stock market, or any other wonderful or pleasant thing you can conceive of in your life. It also comes from losing your job, having difficult deadlines to meet, physical illness, canceled plans, any misfortune, or other negative things you may experience. It is inevitable, but that doesn't mean it's impossible to deal with stress.

If stress is there, what can you do to *manage it? Take stress out of the driver's seat because you can't take it out of your life.* It's always going to be there for the ride.

The Social Readjustment Rating Scale

Psychologists have determined that stress comes from both the positive and the negative things that happen in our lives. In fact, there's a stress scale called the Social Readjustment Rating Scale, also known as the Holmes-Rahe Stress Scale, which provides stress measures for events that can take place in someone's life.

You are asked to note how many of the things have happened to you *in the last 12 months* and then you add up the score. The original research was conducted using a sample of sailors who had been at sea for several months. This makes for a very good study because the factors that could affect the result are experienced by everyone in the study.

Even this scale, however, is only an inadequate and incomplete look at stress and at some of the factors that the authors of the scale believed affected people's physical health. These psychiatrists never provided an exhaustive listing, but rather a broad-stroke approach to the concept of stress and life adjustment.

No attempt should be made to use it as a clinical measure, but it can serve as a guideline for considering the relative impact of stress in life events and how each may affect health. The complete test (see Appendix A), which was constructed to evaluate a 1-year period in someone's life and how stress related to physical illness, has 43 items and is scored as follows:

300 or over: at risk of illness

151–299: moderate risk of illness

150 or less: slight risk of illness

What are some of the items on the scale and what would be given a high value on this scale? Here are just a few examples.

Event	Stress Value
Death of a spouse	100
Divorce	73
Personal injury or illness	53
Marriage	50
Retirement	45
Change in family member's health	44
Pregnancy	40
Business readjustment	39
Change in financial status	38

As you can see, some of these are rather negative stressors and others may be either negative or positive. For example, marriage shouldn't be negative, and neither is retirement or pregnancy, but in each case, there's a *dramatic change in someone's role and responsibilities* and each carries a number of unknowns with it. Change in work responsibilities could mean a job promotion, a change in location, or a cutting back to more reasonable job demands or even having your hours cut.

There are even values placed on changes in sleeping habits (16), vacations (13), Christmas season (12), change in religious activities (19), change in school, residence, or work hours/conditions (all 20), and revision in personal habits (24). The scale also has a value for "outstanding personal achievement" and that's given a point value of 28. Have a great achievement or get fired from your job (47), and you get points either way. Even if the number of family gatherings has been changed (15), there's a value placed on that.

Whichever way you turn, *there are values placed on major events in your life* and, as we've said before, it's not the events, but the way you handle them and how you react that counts. No one needs a master of business administration degree to learn how to manage them, but everyone needs a bit of help in putting it all into a different, more favorable light.

Several of the items on the scale easily fit into the uncertainty brought on by chronic illness in a family. These include the following:

1. The illness
2. Business adjustments
3. Change in financial status
4. Marital arguments
5. Work responsibilities
6. Living conditions, change in residence
7. Work hours, working conditions
8. Social activities
9. Eating habits
10. Change in personal habits

All of these items may relate to multiple sclerosis (MS) in several ways. The disease may cause, as we've seen, cognitive changes that may result in changes in career options, changes in the number of hours you work or the type of work you do, less desire to socialize, change in sleep patterns and finances, or, in some cases, a change of residence. Adding all your values up gives you an approximation of how much stress you're under. Knowing this may help you to redirect and reorder your priorities and make needed change to better deal with these changed demands.

Therefore, it is important to understand that *stress will always be a part of our lives because there is no such thing as "eliminating" stress in our lives.* To experience stress is to be human and we would want nothing less. Stress is emotional and we are emotional creatures but emotions require restraint, too.

It is up to us to learn how to effectively handle or cope with any or all of the stress and to put it, as it were, into perspective in the larger framework of our lives, to see the options, the opportunities, and the challenges. This is especially true for people with MS, where stress plays an extremely important role. Its contribution to the effective functioning of the immune system has been noted by numerous research articles and eminent neurologists.

So, next time you hear someone telling you that you have to get rid of all that stress in your life, you can come back with a realistic response. Perhaps you can help begin a dialogue that will enable them to have a better understanding of the role of stress in all our lives. *There is no such thing as no stress.*

In Chapter 5, we discussed several ways to engage in self-help techniques to lessen, release, or more effectively cope with stress where we have little control over it. Remember, there are always things you can do and you are not helpless. The methods that you choose may not always be able to provide you with all of the relief that you seek, but they can provide some relief.

Consider it a way of putting money in a health account that only you have access to and where you have decided to put just a bit in the bank each day. Slowly building on the account can provide a pleasant surprise when you see how it has grown over the year. I understand that settling for less will not be terribly appealing but even a small change can be a healthy change. Keep as a new inspirational phrase for yourself: *Always look for the possible.* Yes, another refrigerator posting here might be useful as a constant reminder.

One of the first things that you will want to do is to begin to take a very detailed look at your life, your activities, and the demands that are made of you in your various roles.

Stress/Resolution List

Step 1: Take a plain sheet of paper on which the vertical headings will be the *roles* in which you now engage and the horizontal headings are the *stressors* and what you can do to manage it a bit better. I've provided eight roles (patient, spouse, parent, family member, employee, student, consumer, and neighbor) here, but you may have more and your list will be as long as you need.

For example, one role is as a patient. The patient role can involve quite a few stressors and might need a bit more room on your chart. Don't hold back. Write down whatever you feel needs to be addressed in that role, where the stress is experienced, and who or what is the focal point.

Is your physician not understanding you, a health care tech not listening to you, office staff making poorly scheduled appointments, or are there problems with insurance reimbursement or rehab problems? Do you or your spouse need to talk about things in the home, your relationship, or socializing? Is your boss not realizing the need for some changes in your job, where you sit, or something else in the office? I knew one man who had a seat that placed him directly in the sunshine all day long. It was uncomfortable and hot, and he had to speak up to get his desk changed, but it wasn't easy because he didn't want to "make waves" in the office.

It's your list. You don't have to show it to anyone and you can amend it as you wish. Reorder the roles if one appears to need more attention than the others and don't be afraid to shuffle those around, too. The list may constantly be in flux and that's okay because things change.

As you begin to address the stressors and manage in a new, more effective manner, you may find that the number of stressors is decreasing. Part of this may be attributed not only to your willingness to address them but also to your increasing ability to use the "interviewing" skills we've provided in this book. You have become a more effective communicator and you can advocate for yourself. There will be change that you've brought about on your own by your increasing ability to initiate new skills into your fulfillment of many of your roles. *Give yourself credit for this.*

At first, you may not think there's much stress that needs attention in your life and that's not unusual. I knew a young business executive who was under an enormous amount of job stress and had a new baby on the way but he appeared to be handling it quite well until he felt a skipped pulse beat one day. I was in his office that day and he asked me to check his pulse. I'm not a medical doctor, but I did take first aid seminars at hospitals where I had worked. Sure enough, there was a skip and we discussed what he might do about it.

177

Within a week, he was in a yoga stress-management group on his lunch hour and practicing both exercising daily and relaxation breathing. Two months more and the pulse beat was back to normal. But first, his body had to tell him that something was amiss before he took action. Your stress may not show up as a skipped beat, but it will manifest itself in some respect, whether physical or emotional.

Other areas of major concern for your chart might be your job, your school, or some other activity and another might be your role as a parent or partner. Across the top of the chart you are constructing, have at least three vertical columns: **My Roles, Stressors**, and **Resolution**.

My Roles	Stressors	Resolution
Patient		
Spouse		
Parent		
Family member		
Employee		
Student		
Consumer		
Neighbor		

Step 2: Jot down a few words that describe the stress you experience *in each role* in the **Stressors** column.

Take a moment out right now to consider each of your roles here. I'll start off with a few examples of areas where there might be stress and you can use these as jumping-off points for your own list.

Patient: appointment scheduling, medication instructions, forms needed, refills, insurance forms, handicapped parking, hours of operation, callbacks from health care staff, payments schedules, waiting time in the office

Spouse: household chores, finances, shopping, socializing, appointments, recreational opportunities, in-laws, transportation, job responsibilities

Parent: parental needs, visits, holidays, assistance with household or financial matters, vacations, travel, medical needs

Family member: sibling relationships, visiting, communication, assistance, information regarding MS, and treatments. Some of the most problematic here are when families get together for holidays. Going over what happened last year and how to handle it if it happens again this year might be a good idea. Anticipation is not just a "Carly Simon song."

Employee: hours of work, job site, duties, compensation, location, access to office, office setup, time off, sick leave, insurance, questions of accommodation for MS patients, human resources policies

Student: testing accommodation, campus travel, counseling, class absences, student aid, class location, makeup policy, tutoring, incompletes policy, classroom seating

Consumer: You are a consumer not only when you go to the store, shop online, go down to the gas station, or your child's school but also when you receive health care services and products. In each of these roles where you purchase a service or item, you have an interaction that can be pleasant, informative, or difficult.

How have your consumer interactions been lately? See any need for a change here? In stores, the interaction may be set up in a negatively skewed fashion, as it was when I heard a store manager approach a dissatisfied customer with the question, "What's the problem here?" Suppose it had been phrased, "How can I help you?" It would have made a world of difference by just taking that word *problem* out and putting in the word *help*.

Neighbor: Neighbors can be the people who live next door, down the block, or who sit in the next cubicle from you at work. They can even be the people sitting near you on a plane, train, bus, or in a car. *The stressor can be the physically close relationship and this may be troublesome because it invades your personal space* in some way; sometimes physically, sometimes by how people conduct themselves in their choice of music or entertainment, or by their lack of social graces. Neighbors can almost be like members of your family because you may feel stuck with them, not by birth, but by real estate choice or job location.

Step 3: At this step is where you consider each stressor and come up with *some way you can try to manage that stress a bit better*. What other stressors can you find here or what was sparked by this listing? Make your list as items occur to you; put items in the margins of this book. Highlighting is definitely permitted in this book and, in fact, encouraged.

If nothing comes to mind right away, that's okay. Come back to it when something does pop up in your mind and jot it down. Post it where you'll be sure to see it until it is almost filled. Understand that you can revise this list regarding the stress and the resolution, and it's another one of those *works in progress* I've been talking about in this book.

The Gentle Art of Persuasion

One thing that people in sales have to learn quickly and learn well is to be an effective communicator, but more than that, they need to learn to be persuasive. Bringing someone to their point of view about a product or service means they are going to get what they want—the sale.

You may not be engaged in anything like sales, but you do need to adopt the skills of a salesperson because you do want to get things done, you want to bring people around to seeing your point of view, and you want to get along well with others. Remember that neighbor you may have problems with and who was causing a bit of stress in your life? What about that person who didn't seem to understand your medical coverage or when you were disputing a charge or you wanted a copy of something? Do you think one of those cases might have benefitted from *a bit more in the gentle art of persuasion*?

One man, Dale Carnegie, wrote a simple "how to" book in 1937 and the book is still going strong and being used by corporations all over the world. In fact, the book is used in professional training seminars and public speaking courses. It was his premise that people like to be appreciated and given credit for things, even if they didn't come up with the idea in the first place. This tactic helped Carnegie sell 15 million books.

Persuasion, therefore, is 85% of what Carnegie saw as the simple task of expressing *yourself well and arousing enthusiasm in others*. In other words, make them feel important and you're on your way to the "sale." The word *sale* may sound a bit crass, I agree, but you do have to sell yourself constantly in various settings and once you make that sale, things will go much smoother for you in the future.

One of your first steps in the persuasion process is simple: smile. Smiles have a way of providing a visual sign that you want to be agreeable, that you're not an enemy, and that you seek a pleasant encounter with them. If you have a problem, perhaps a bit of preparation just before the encounter is a good idea.

Just pull back a bit, help yourself to compose your thoughts and begin with that smile. A compliment, simple pleasantries, and relaxed body language helps, too. How do you suppose all those politicians get elected in the first place? They smile even when they're being criticized bitterly. They agree that the other person has a good point in their argument and they admit that they can see their point of view. They even talk about their own mistakes and how they felt either foolish or angry or at a loss for words. See how they present themselves as being just as human as you? Pedestals are for statues; people need to have their feet on the ground and admit they have had a stumble or two. When you do that, you're letting the other person know you share things in common.

Persuasion also depends on that interviewing skill I talked about earlier. You establish rapport by tossing away all those "whys" and beginning to use both restatement and personal disclosure. Once you've done that, you will notice a change in things.

You already know that you'll have to have all the facts about whatever you need to discuss and to have considered the possible comments to each of your points. Prepare how you will answer these comments in an agreeable manner. Above all, keep those emotions in check. If you are having a problem there, pull out those relaxation breathing exercises and begin to give yourself a good 5 minutes or so to calm down even before the interaction begins.

Some things you also want to look out for, which I discuss in the next few paragraphs, are those *automatic thoughts* that cause so many people problems. Read that section carefully and check to see where you may need a little work.

Quality of Life

One of the things I'd like to discuss in this portion of the book is the quality of your life and what that will mean to you in terms of MS and your ability to handle it. Stress resolution that you've just begun to note on the previous table is part of this because how you feel and how you react to things spreads out into your life like ripples on a pond.

You know that when things aren't going well with your MS or with your family, your job, or your friends, you can get pretty down. Add that to the cognitive challenges of MS and it's not easy to do the things you must. Those are the days you'd rather pull up the covers and stay in bed all day.

To help you take a more definitive look at various aspects of your life and your level of satisfaction or dissatisfaction with them, we've provided a self-scoring scale (see Appendix B) in the back of the book. We've chosen this particular scale because it was designed to be used by persons who have chronic medical illnesses. Review it, rate the items in the scale, and look at your score. What does it tell you or what did the scale point out to you? This scale fits in very well with the question of roles and how the demands of each and the resolution of problems has an impact on you.

We haven't provided scoring because the scale is meant solely to act as a means of helping you view your current feelings about your life. The higher your number on any item on the scale and the higher your total score, without a doubt, mean that you are very satisfied and happy. However, don't view this in any way other than as an index regarding where you may want to make changes and where you may have skipped over an important aspect of your life right now. Give it some thought.

What does research have to do with your roles and how you function in them? It's one way for me to help you see what can be done, if you will keep on going and getting others in your life to help. I'm talking about relationships and what they mean to your physical and mental health.

A chronic illness brings with it many challenges, but no one has to tell you that. You already know it. However, staying involved has a great deal to do with remaining healthy, and your family, friends, and acquaintances have a lot to do with it, too. They are, in effect, like the medicine you take without needing a prescription.

Consider your roles and how much responsibility you are required to exercise in each. What gives you pleasure in each of these roles and what causes you difficulty or stress? You are now beginning to identify the areas of stress in each of the roles and, once identified, you can begin to consider possible ways to amend the role or the stress level.

Also, as you consider your roles, do something that therapists look for during therapy sessions: *look for automatic thoughts*. These are thoughts that you immediately use, almost without thinking, whenever something happens to you in your life. Are they negative thoughts? They may well be and that's something you are about to change.

What comes to your mind, automatically, when something problematic happens? Think about it. How is this helpful? Is it helpful? I think you might be surprised at what you find. The way you respond has a great impact on the quality of your relationships and those relationships can mean a great deal to you, so you want to work at maintaining them. Who wants to be around someone who is always seeing the negative in life or who never has a kind word or thinks that the sky is falling?

Let me give you a simple example of someone who had come to my attention at one time. She was a young woman who had a history of cancer, but was stabilized now and doing quite well. She was in a therapist's office for her regular appointment and had told her therapist that she was very upset.

The therapist asked what the problem was. She answered that she'd have to buy a new car and she couldn't afford it. What made her think she had to buy a new car? It seemed that her car was making noise now and she was convinced it couldn't be fixed. She'd have to buy a new one. Had she talked to a mechanic? No, but she knew what the answer would be. How did she know the answer if she wasn't a mechanic? She just knew.

It was an example of *catastrophizing*: thinking the worst possible thing when other alternatives were available, but hidden from her ability to see them. She was engaging in a type of automatic thinking. The therapist discussed her concerns with her, her feelings of financial ruin if she had to buy a new car, the fact that she needed a car, and her inability to get one.

What could she do? They decided what she needed to do was to consult a mechanic and get an idea of what was wrong with the car and whether it could be fixed. She did and the mechanic said it needed a muffler. When she realized it wasn't as bad as she had thought, the sun came out in the sky for her again and she smiled. It was only a muffler she needed!

I know you're not concerned with cars, but you get the point. Begin to look at the other side of things and *see the possible rather than the problem*. Have you ever caught yourself catastrophizing? How did you resolve the problem?

Before we go on to your roles in your life, let's take a short detour to outline some simple ways to get things back on track whenever they go awry. These are just a few things that will be helpful in juggling all your roles.

Learning "Interviewing" Skills

Looking at this heading, you may be wondering how "interviewing" fits into this chapter or even this book because it's not about careers. Yes, it is. It's about your life as a career, which you have to manage every day and where interviewing skills are going to be one of your strongest assets.

You have goals in mind (probably to be as happy as possible) and you need to make plans to get there just as you would in career planning. Handling other people, whether in an office or a home, depends on much the same skills, which aren't beyond your abilities.

The following are two of the most important things you can do:

1. Avoid the use of "why" and try to find another way to ask a question.
2. It's okay to state a problem using what are called "I" messages where you state the reasons you are having a problem. I'll explain why "you" have the problem in a minute.

What happens when you phrase a question beginning with "why"? Simple. You put the other person on the defensive and you don't create a situation where understanding and compromise (very important) can be achieved. What is your objective? Do you want to "win" here or get some resolution or help? "Winning" will gain you only a short-lived sense of being "right" and then what?

You want to be satisfied that you're being heard and you want to know that both of you will be able to continue in a working relationship. This is particularly important when it comes to working with your health care professionals or your family, coworkers, and friends.

I've heard people say that their physicians aren't listening to them or not providing enough information to them. If that's the case, how can you resolve that problem? You shouldn't be expected to understand everything about your disorder if it's phrased in medical lingo, so ask for a simpler explanation. If you don't ask and forget about using that "why" format, you won't get the answers you need. You're not a physician, you may not know what certain words mean, but that doesn't mean you are dumb, ill-informed, or can't understand. Yes, you can understand if it is restated in simpler terms.

Remember, too, that it's okay to use "I" statements where you state how you feel so that someone understands more fully. If you're feeling confused about a conversation you're having about something, say your treatment options or consequences, let the other person know. If you don't let them know, they can't respond appropriately and that just keeps the confusion going. Clear it up and you can move on. The relationship will definitely benefit from this simple rule, but remember, you have to take that step back and use that rephrasing and "I" method to do it.

The Four Accusations

Let's take a look at some of the ways you can use statements that point toward the other person as the culprit and how using an "I" statement instead might help in smoothing things out.

Have you found yourself using one or all of the following statements:

1. "You are making me so mad."
2. "You are a (fill in the blanks with negative words here) . . ."
3. "I'm so angry I could just (fill in the blanks) . . ." or "You had better (fill in the blanks) . . ."
4. "You don't know what you're talking about."

Do any of them sound familiar to you? Turn it around a bit and look at the first statement. We'll take each of the statements in turn and give you a quick view of what may be actually communicated here.

How Each Accusation Can Be Viewed

Accusation No. 1 is untrue because *only you* can "make" you mad. You are feeling mad because of something that happened, so why not explain what that is and how you were interpreting it?

Accusation No. 2 can be seen as an opportunity to state how you feel about a person's actions and how they affected you or made you feel. Name calling, as the old children's rhyme states, inaccurately, *will hurt both you and the person with whom you're trying to interact.* Take the opportunity, whenever this happens, to remain silent until you can collect your thoughts and express yourself in a more cooperative manner. These types of statements are highly judgmental and will raise anyone's back in reactive anger.

Accusation No. 3 is one I see as being "loaded for bear" and it's a serious mistake to begin to make these types of statements. They usually carry with them an intention of taking some action that you will regret later because *they are, in a way, a threat.*

Accusation No. 4 is when you state you don't think they know what they're talking about and why is that? How did you come to that conclusion? Do they not understand what you've said? Are they assuming something they shouldn't? Do you need to supply more information to them? I find this is usually the case when you haven't had a chance to really help them understand what you're going through. Then, perhaps, they would know what they were talking about.

Don't just engage in a verbal knee-jerk response like this; say how you feel about what they're indicating. True, they may not know what they're talking about, especially if it concerns how bad you feel that day or how your illness is affecting you and your quality of life. The answer here is to open up the discussion instead of shutting the door with pronouncements like this.

Restatement is one of the most effective methods therapists use in working with anyone and it's something you can use, too. When you do this, stating back to someone what they've just said, they understand that you are following them and it keeps the conversation going. If your restatement is off the mark, they can tell you and begin a fuller explanation of what they meant.

You might also use, "Help me to understand what you mean here," and then give a shortened version of what they said *as you heard it.* Notice I said, *as you heard it?* That's because we each interpret what we're hearing *through the filter of our experience and expectations,* so it's not always what the other person meant at all. Expectancy on your part has a lot to do with what you "hear" or fail to hear.

Choosing the least negative, most collaborative response to something will do quite a lot to dampen those fires of depression and anxiety that may be burning within you. It surely will take some practice and effort on your part when you find yourself about to blurt something out without first stopping for a few seconds to consider the content and the reaction you'll get.

It's all part of being a more effective communicator and that's half the battle in life. Count to three in your mind, if that will help. This way you have a bit of time to hold back that initial, perhaps too emotional, response and to formulate something a bit more helpful to your cause. If at all possible, try to smile, as I said before. No, not everyone feels like smiling, but it helps.

Your Role as Your Medical Advocate

Take a look at your role as your own medical advocate. You interact with several health care professionals who provide services to you, perhaps tests, medications, some form of physical or mental therapy, help with obtaining insurance, or other kinds of services you may need. What is most stressful for you in any of these situations? There may be some situations that are more stressful than others are, but just go back to that list I mentioned before and start writing down what you find most stressful. Now, reorder your list for your "patient" role from top to bottom with the top item being the most stressful and the bottom being the least stressful. You've now got the stressors there and you can work on the resolutions.

Communication with your health care providers is extremely important in everything, including health outcomes. One of the results found in a research study with women who had breast cancer was that those who maintained effective communication with their treating physicians had better outcomes. So, communication was the essential factor in creating an emotional and physical environment, which contributed to successful treatment outcomes. These women were also more optimistic about their outcomes postsurgery.

This isn't a book about cancer or women with cancer, but studies such as this can provide insights into how patients and medical staff can both contribute in intangible ways to successful treatment. It's the same with MS. The words used and the freely exchanged concerns and considerations all point to benefits for all. How a person is treated and how sensitivity and respect are shown are also crucial for positive communication.

I'll provide an example of something I witnessed in a medical setting. A woman had to have a heart monitoring procedure and the technician was a woman. The technician told the woman to undress to the waist, put on a robe with the opening in the front, and lie down on the table. She was very uncomfortable getting undressed in front of the technician and asked her to leave. "Why should I leave?—we're both women," she responded.

The woman was quite angry, but felt intimidated and complied. Later, however, she was angry both at the technician and at herself for not speaking up and asking, firmly, that the technician leave. The physician, who was reading the test results, noted that her blood pressure (BP) was elevated and he expressed concern. The woman indicated what had happened and they took the BP again. It was lower, but not back to her normal reading.

Should the woman have complied without complaint or did she have a valid request that wasn't honored? It didn't matter that they were both women; one of them wasn't respecting the other and a medical test reading, as a result, was altered.

Identify what you believe causes the stress in each of your role categories. Perhaps you feel that you are not being heard when you talk about one of your symptoms, which has been distressing for you. Go over the interviewing skills I just outlined. You may feel that you are not being given the time you need to fully participate in some form of therapy. Maybe you don't understand the instruction that you were given regarding medication or therapy. Prior to coming to the therapy you may have been feeling a bit rushed, and it is this rushed feeling that may be spilling over into the therapy.

You may also have been feeling that there was a problem with your memory and, if the therapist gave you instructions, you may have felt you were being treated poorly or not in a respectful manner. Instead of helping you remember the instructions, you just heard what you hadn't understood before all over again. You still didn't understand and it was stressful.

How did you respond to this feeling of being rushed or of having problems remembering the instructions? Can you ask for instructions to be written out or to be left at the front desk for you to pick up as you leave? How can this situation be made more comfortable for you? Should you bring someone with you, record the instructions on your tape, or write them down? The decision is yours as to what you do here, but you play a part in reducing the tension.

These are just some examples of things that you may have experienced. I'm sure you can think of other instances where you had a problem in an interaction and went away feeling angry, anxious, or depressed as a result.

You may have heard yourself using those old, "I should have . . ." or "Why didn't I . . .?" statements. How helpful is that now?

It's not useful, so what's the reason to keep going over it? The future is where you aim and next time you can reshape the interaction.

Once you've identified the cause, you can begin to consider what you can do to reduce that stress. For instance, if you feel that there is an individual with whom you must regularly interact and who causes you a great deal of stress, is there a possibility that you can make them aware of this in an acceptable manner? I believe this can be done, but you may want to have some support with you when you approach this topic. It's always a good idea to have a support person not only who can help facilitate certain interactions, but who will be there to remember what took place and what was agreed on or to help get clarification of something. Just because you didn't go to medical school or get a graduate school education, doesn't mean you can't understand something. Yes, you can and they have a responsibility to help you understand.

Any treatment for your MS may evoke anxiety and stress. One thing that can help is when you have a sense of control and also the ability to express your needs and concerns. You want people to work with you in a helpful manner and I'm sure they want to do the same, but they can't if you haven't made them aware of your difficulties.

Clearing up any misconceptions is part of the solution and you will be able to do this. You can ask to have any procedure explained in advance, know who will or is performing it, and decide if you're comfortable with the procedure and/or the person. I think everyone, upon meeting a new patient, should introduce himself or herself and indicate what they are going to do for you. Not everyone adheres to that policy and not everyone wears a tag telling you his or her job title.

I once heard a rather inexperienced physician responding to a patient in a manner that I found unacceptable and I have instructed hundreds of students about this. The patient said she wanted to know more about a specific procedure and the reason why it was to be done before she would agree to it. "I have over 400 patients," the physician said, "and you're the first one who wouldn't do as I asked. I'm your doctor and *you have to listen to me.*"

The patient, fortunately, had a relative in the room who agreed that there would have to be mutual agreement before there was any action taken on a procedure. The physician was informed, in a very civil manner, that this was a collaborative effort, not one where he alone made the decisions. For many people, the white coat syndrome is still strong and it's often difficult to stand up when there's a dilemma.

Let me give you one small piece of advice that I have always given to both my therapy patients and the thousands of college and medical students I've taught over the years. If there is *one word* that you should eliminate from your vocabulary, as I've said before, to have more pleasant and productive interactions with people, that word would be *why*. You've seen how to do this in my interviewing tips previously, but a bit of reinforcement always helps.

Once you say, "why" to someone you begin down a road where it's going to be very bumpy, will take longer than you'd planned, and may not have the outcome you desire. You've undermined your wish to have someone understand and work with you.

Instead of asking "why," before you ever utter a word, work that question around in your mind until it comes out without "why" in it. Try it and see how well it can work for you right now. The next person who crosses your path, try asking the reason they're doing something, but don't use "why." Do this as much as possible over the coming week and you'll become more comfortable with it and it will become second nature.

Okay, you have your homework assignment for the coming week. No more "whys" as much as is humanly possible and every question that would have had a "why" is to be reworked. Instead of "why" you can substitute, "Let's see if I got this right," or "The reason you want to do that is . . ." or maybe, "I guess I should want to (fill in what you think you're supposed to be doing) because . . ."

See how well you do and don't be surprised if things become a lot more pleasant for you. You might even practice this at home before you go anywhere that the "why" question might come up and it can come up a lot in so many places. Don't worry; you will learn to tame this dragon.

Regaining Self-Esteem and Pride

William (see Chapter 3) had to learn his newfound shortcomings in terms of his temper on his own. As he said,

> The first thing that I became aware of, that I was doing to myself, was my own frustration was slowing me down. I was reaching for anger as my only response. Normally, at myself, but it was aimed at anybody near me. You'd wonder why my

flash point seemed to be lowered and easily set off. When you can't do what you did before and that you took for granted, it's difficult and frustrating. It's not as if I used to juggle 16 balls at one time and now I can only juggle 14. No, I mean all of a sudden, you can't juggle at all.

The frustration is that you look to yourself and wander [*sic*], "What did I do?" What did I do to deserve this or what did I do to cause it? I decided I needed to shift that away from blaming myself, which I thought was an excuse not to deal with it. I shifted it to, "What can you do?" Identify what you're doing to make it worse, because you can't stop what's happening. I was told right away there was no cure for MS. Okay, I figured, I'm not going to sit and wait for the cure, but I'm not going to make it worse by beating up on myself, by acting out.

Stress proved to be one place William could act effectively on his own behalf.

The answer for me was that I needed to cut back on stress. I needed to identify what would set me off, my flash points, and how to better deal with that, so I decided to retire, because I didn't want to do any damage to my business relationships with clients. I would have had to disclose my MS to clients. What clients would want someone like that? It just layered the stress on me.

I wanted to cut loose what I was carrying inside of me as far as stress. I felt it would turn into more guilt. I would feel more guilt that I wasn't serving my clients as I should, or guilty that I wasn't being a better husband, a better dad, or whatever it was and I didn't want to layer more invisible stress on top of it.

Retirement and Purpose

Retirement wasn't the end of it all for William; it was a beginning. The beginning came as a new path in his life and this path led him to become more involved in helping others understand and deal with MS. He would become an advocate, a speaker at MS events, and a ready ear for anyone who wanted to share his or her journey and his or her knowledge with others. During this time, he said:

> I continued to work with the neuropsychologist and a lot of it became clear because she had a way of calling it out, as it was happening. She didn't let me try to double talk myself around it, but I was doing that and it was very easy. She would say, "Why are you sitting here?" She would say that, if I were sitting there trying to convince myself or someone else that this is okay and that I didn't have to change, then I didn't need to do it there. She'd tell me that if I wanted to hold on to the vital elements of my life, which meant prioritizing, I was going to have to let go of certain things in my life and decide what's important.

This was when the value of therapy became quickly evident to William.

> She didn't hand me any answers of what to do, but helped me answer it for myself and she held me accountable. She would quote what I had said back to me. She would say, "Well, you said that this was most important." Or, "You said that this was the stress and you were going to try to relieve it, so why are you hanging on to it?" What can you do to delegate it or get some kind of help in something that is vital like doing your family finances or the checkbook, and things like that? You can't just decide not to do that anymore. It was a case of where do I begin to do this?

Decisions had to be made that meant William would have to give up some control over things in his life and that was a difficult issue. "Should I bring in an accountant, another relative, or a friend to help with financial matters? She helped me identify where the weak points were and where else I could help myself to change things."

Change and stress relief didn't come without some discomfort for William. "It was a tremendous ego blow having to ask for help to do that. It's like being a swimmer for your entire life and having someone say to you that they don't want you in the pool, anymore. They tell you they don't want you swimming anymore, and if you are going to get into the pool, you'll need to put on a life vest and you need to let somebody know that you're getting into the pool. You can't do it by yourself.

"You'd feel like a child. I thought that if I enable myself to continue to do certain vital things, it is better for me to decide what I shouldn't do or what I need help with and to delegate, rather than have it yanked from me."

The decisions had to be made himself, not by someone else allocating responsibility to another person.

> I started to think of seniors who have driven for their entire life and then, at one point, their children sit them down and tell them they're going to have to hand their license in. I didn't want to do that. When the cognitive part reared its head, I was only 40 or 41 years old. I didn't want my business taken away. I didn't want clients to turn on me. I didn't want to go sour that way, so I figured I would take a little leadership in it and admit the decision and the difficulties that were there and ask for help.

One point that needed to be addressed, too, was William's sense of loss of purpose, possibly, his need to continue to play a vital role in his own life and to gain a sense of accomplishment. He had been a high achiever all his life and now he needed to find something that would fill that void left when he had to leave his profession.

William chose to volunteer as a way to get involved in life again.

> It's prideful because you feel you're doing something. It's sort of like many careers where you ask someone what you like about it and, whether it's a doctor or nurse, or someone like that, and they say, "I like helping people." I think that as a volunteer I get as much, if not more, out of it than the people who it is supposed to benefit.

Positive Relationships

Psychologists know not only from years of experience, but also from some classic experiments, that anxiety as well as good spirits can be brought about by the people around us. One interviewee stated it this way,

> I noticed that positive energy can be very contagious. Mind your company, stay around good people; energetic, positive people. Anyone who seems to cause frustration can wear on someone. Consider how you can have less interactions with them, but do it in a sensitive way. Unfortunately, some people just rob you of all sorts of energy by their attitude. They bring

you down, especially when they are negative in their outlook and are always critical.

As William had indicated, he found that going out and volunteering was one of the most positive steps anyone could take.

I think it starts with doing positive things, engaging in positive activities, and it can be through volunteer work through the school with your children, with the church, with MS organizations.

I think volunteering is a very important part of staying active, staying involved, staying engaged and you'll find positive people in those places. Wherever there are positive things going on, whether it's at the Y, an exercise club or wherever you go, you're going to find people that are positively engaged somehow, some way.

Discussing Your Diagnosis

As several of the interviewees indicated, there is still a belief that a diagnosis of MS carries with it a trace of stigma. Sarah, in her characteristic fashion, chose to meet the challenge head on and approach it in an open fashion. However, she understands how it may be difficult for anyone who has had little contact with someone with MS and, therefore, little knowledge about it. They just don't know how to respond and it can cause initial discomfort for both parties.

Keeping positive and maintaining positive relationships and a sense of self-worth were all important to Sarah, as they are to anyone with or without a chronic illness. She chose to tell whomever she wished, didn't hide it, and went on with her life much as she had before. Sarah had seen what could happen if someone decided to keep his or her MS a secret and shape his or her life around this secret. Remember the fellow who hadn't dated in 10 years? Not discussing his diagnosis had put him into a limbo in terms of dating and socializing and he tried desperately to hide it. The energy that must have taken to do that was just unfathomable, as Sarah saw it.

Maintaining positive relationships was an important thread that ran through all the interviews conducted for this book and, rather than interpret what they said, I've allowed them to speak for themselves in expressing their thoughts.

Not everyone is in a work setting, some of the interviewees are retired for one reason or another, but all of them maintain social relationships where their illness has come up at various times. All of them have formed a support system composed of family, friends, neighbors, and coworkers in addition to contacts in local MS groups.

Whether it's just going for coffee with her friends, as Anna had said, her friends seemed to understand she could talk to them easily about her MS and how it affected her life. Anna encouraged anyone with MS to find their friends and talk to them. She has found their support and understanding bolster her ability to deal with any problems her MS may cause.

Retrieving Good From Bad

As William had discovered, "I didn't want to hurt people and close relatives and friends. When you tell some people that you have MS and they tear up and start crying right in front of you, uncontrollably, it's as if you asked them to come to your funeral. What that said to me was that there was an opportunity there to help them understand what this really means." He now understood how little education there had been for people without MS and how this led to beliefs that were out of line with the current state of treatment.

It was a time for education and, once William realized that he had MS and that was a fact of life, he also began to see that he could do something about it and turn this around.

> Whatever they think they've heard or know about MS, they need to be updated because, yes, I've known people who have died from complications of MS, but they are far and few between. A lot of that may have to do with age, when they were diagnosed, when the medication became available and on and on and on.

> The MS we have now is not the MS of 30 years ago. So there is good news and bad news. The bad news is you have MS, but the good news is that this is a great time to deal with it.

> People outside the MS community needed education and to know that there was more that they could do besides pity me or anyone with MS. Honestly, I didn't want their pity. Sympathy doesn't really do anything for me or anybody else who has MS. But if we can turn that into getting them to participate in something like an MS walk, then that's being active.

195

The many activities in the MS community have included both MS walks and MS bike rides.

> For the past few years, we've had a record number of about 70 people on our team for the MS walk. People say they are sorry to hear I have MS and they'll throw in that, 'If there's anything I can do,' and I will jump in and thank them for offering and tell them about a fundraiser we're having or there's a silent auction coming up, whatever. There's so much to do. For instance, it will be a luncheon they can sponsor and on and on. So if they mean it, and they usually do, I'm going to put something into their hands that will give them something to do.

His enthusiasm and energy are contagious and it's hard not to hear that coming across as he discusses the many things that *can* be done with regard to MS and finding a cure or funds for research or any other MS-related activity.

Roger and Sarah, too, are enthusiastic about the MS bike rides. As Roger said,

> Why are certain "adjustments" seen as positive and acceptable while others are seen as negative and "giving up"? How can modifying our approach to how we do things be viewed as positive in one area of life yet negative in others? If I alter my approach and make necessary adaptation to "stay in the game," isn't that positive, no matter the conditions or circumstances?

Roger made the decision that if he couldn't participate in the MS bike ride on a regular two-wheeler, he'd find another way and he did. It was another opportunity to use his problem-solving skills.

"This year, I rode 40 miles of the MS150 in a recumbent trike. I began considering a trike last season as I was having difficulties holding myself up on a two-wheeled bike. The decision to purchase a new bike did not come easy. It was expensive, I already owned a bike and the money could have been used elsewhere."

However, there was another consideration for Roger.

> Another part of the anguish I put myself through stems from my own unwillingness to give up and this is (was) my own mental block that needed adjusting. I was falling. I had experienced several near misses with cars, ditches and trees all while

riding my regular, two-wheeler street bike. I valued the fresh air while exercising, I valued the MS150 and our team. In time, out of necessity, I began to view a trike as a way to stay in the game and I love it. It offers me the security of steadiness much in the same way my cane assists me while walking. The key term here is "assists"!

The trike solution, for Roger, was enlivening and it lifted his mood whenever he had a chance to ride the new trike. No longer a sign of his inability to bike ride, it was a sign of his resilience and resolution to make changes.

Sarah is very enthusiastic about the MS bike ride in her city.

The day I found out I had MS, I cried, I was upset, but I had to learn how to channel my feelings. I went to work, I did all the things I had to and I went out shopping on my lunch hour. Anything, to make myself feel better and I even signed up for an MS Society bike ride. The coolest thing was that after I signed up for the bike ride and got my team and we were in the event, we ended up raising over $5,000!

What the bike ride did for me also was that it really amazed me how many people came out to help. Some of them I hadn't had contact with for years; people I didn't even know that well wanted to be on my team. For me, I guess, it was just an affirmation of the goodness of people and that's something that you can kind of forget because of the other stuff in your life.

Attitude Is Everything

The one theme that runs through all of the interviewees' statements about themselves and the actions they took has to be a prime example of positive psychology in action. Despite their circumstances, their age differences, or the state of their MS, all of them found ways in which they could make both large and small changes in their lives, which would be acceptable and realistic.

None of them felt their fate was hopeless, or that they could not accommodate to their MS. They are, in effect, true believers of the premise that Dr. Seligman expounds in his books. They saw what they could change and what they couldn't, and they took action.

In the true pioneering spirit that allowed people to venture forth into uncharted waters, these men and women are "bootstrappers." They didn't wait for anyone to pull them along; they pulled themselves up. I use this metaphor, because in this portion of the journey, despite a considerable body of research and incredible efforts regarding this disease, the waters are still uncharted.

The concept of helplessness has been explored in both Dr. Seligman's book and research articles. In the research, it has been shown that a *sense of helplessness effectively contributes to feelings of fatigue and depression in MS patients*. Fatigue was not seen as caused by depression alone, and it was suggested that helplessness was an important factor in feelings of fatigue. This bolstered the belief that there is a direct relationship between how patients feel about themselves and their abilities and their lack of energy as well as low self-esteem.

If, as some people say, "attitude is everything," then you know where you have to go and what you have to do.

Maintaining Hope

A proverb by an unknown Turkish writer instructs us that, "Things never go so well that one should have no fear, and never so ill that one should have no hope." Hope is the one thing that can make the unbearable bearable once again because it provides the promise that the future holds many bits of serendipity for us, not just tribulations.

Writing for those who had reason to find hope in short supply, Thomas Jefferson, one of the truly great minds of the past 200 years, said, "When you reach the end of your rope, tie a knot in it and hang on." Hang on, don't give up, don't allow yourself to fall off, but be inventive and see that even in the direst of situations, there is hope. Put that one on your refrigerator door, too, and print it in large, bold letters.

Seligman, too, writes that, "Once you recognize that you have a pessimistic thought that seems unwarranted, argue against it using the ABCDE model." He outlines what that stands for as:

A: adversity—yes, it may be bad, but are you catastrophizing?

B: beliefs that come automatically

C: consequences that come from these beliefs

D: disputation of these knee-jerk beliefs

E: energization that comes from fighting those beliefs

In going through this simple routine, Seligman offers a quick way to help you rebalance and maintain your sense of hope in the face of often-difficult times in your life. Things aren't going to be as they always have been, living is reaching for the possible and the potential and, yes, there are silver linings in some of those clouds. Notice I didn't say *all* because a dose of pragmatism should be used prudently in everything you do.

Because I've provided several inspirational proverbs and comments from others, let me leave you with one from my ancestors:

May the road rise up to meet you,

May the wind be ever at your back.

May the sun shine warm upon your face and rain fall softly on your field.

Further Reading

Beaton D. Effects of stress and psychological disorders on the immune system. 2003. Available at: www.personalityresearch.org/papers/beaton.html. Accessed September 14, 2010.

Brown RF, Tennant CC, Sharrock M, Hodgkinson S, et al. Relationship between stress and relapse in multiple sclerosis: Part 1. Important features. *Mult Scler*, 2006;12(4):453–464.

Carnegie D. *How to Win Friends and Influence People*. New York: Simon & Schuster; 2009.

Gold SM, Mohr DC, Huitinga I, Flachenecker P, et al. The role of stress-response systems for the pathogenesis and progression of MS. *Trends Immunol*, 2005;26(12). Available at: http://www.direct-ms.org/pdf/ImmunologyMS/GoldStressMS.pdf. Accessed September 14, 2010.

Holmes TH, Rahe R H. The Social Readjustment Rating Scale. *J Psychosom Res*, 1967;11(2):213–218.

Seligman MEP. *What You Can Change . . . and What You Can't: The Complete Guide to Successful Self-Improvement*. New York: Ballantine Books; 1993.

Seligman MEP. *Authentic Happiness: Using the New Positive Psychology to Realize Your Potential for Lasting Fulfillment*. New York: Free Press; 2002.

Van der Werf SP, Evers A, Jongen PJ, Bleijenberg G. The role of helplessness as mediator between neurological disability, emotional instability, experienced fatigue and depression in patients with multiple sclerosis. *Mult Scler*, 2003;9(1):89–94.

9

The Future Is Bright

Change is in the air for important, even dramatic, advances in research and treatments for multiple sclerosis (MS) and that is the message we hope to provide for our readers. Anyone with a diagnosis of MS is living in the best of times because of the vigorous attention now being paid to find new treatments for MS.

The goals are many and Dr. Jeffrey Cohen, director of Mellen Center Experimental Therapeutics, Cleveland Clinic, is very optimistic about current developments and future research.

> If I were speaking to MS patients, I'd say that, in general, our understanding of the disease has advanced year by year, including causative factors, how the damage occurs in MS, how to measure the damage and which things may modify how much damage accumulates.
>
> Secondly, one of the important issues is our ability to predict how someone is going to respond to various medications.

That aspect of treatment, according to Dr. Cohen, "is something where we're really making some headway and, in terms of the types of treatments, this can relieve some of the anxiety associated with the disease's unpredictable nature."

Looking forward, Dr. Cohen sees many new medications currently in clinical trials and, as a result, even further advances in treatment options. "On a hopeful note, there are seven medications approved by regulatory agencies to treat the disease and there are a sizeable number of new medications on the horizon."

One of the main advantages of the new medications is in the method of administration. "About half of the new treatments are oral and this addresses one of the issues with the current medications which are all taken by injection. The new treatments have fewer side effects, too, and appear to be more effective." The whole issue of having to deal with daily injections has presented drawbacks for patients who have had difficulty with injectables. Patients have been reluctant to learn the technique because of their anxiety and fears related to injections. This concern has led to efforts by specially trained nurses who are conducting sessions to help patients deal with this aspect of their daily treatment regime. It is felt that a pill would both clear the way for a more readily acceptable administration of the med and raise levels of compliance.

"Finally, all of the medications I've just talked about are largely preventative so their job is to keep things from getting worse, but they don't restore function when there's already been damage. We are, however, finally starting to move into a phase where we're evaluating strategies for improving function." Some of the new and very promising treatments include work with stem cell applications. These have proved to be helpful in other diseases and immune disorders, and the hope is that they will also be useful in MS where it may be possible to effect regeneration where damage has occurred.

Anxiety and depression, Dr. Cohen admitted, have been problems associated with not only the anxiety surrounding the disorder, but also the biological underpinnings of MS. The new medications aimed at MS itself may also, indirectly, bring about an improvement in anxiety, depression, and resulting mood shifts.

> We've come to realize that some of the anxiety and depression is biological in addition to the reaction to receiving this diagnosis and the possibility of disability. We do have a sense that even people who are doing pretty well and whose disease appears stable still exhibit a higher incidence of depression, probably related to the biology of the disease.

A new, preliminary study at the Cleveland Clinic was, at the time of writing of this book, about 4 months away from initiation.

> We have a preliminary study on stem cells that is about to get started. I think stem cells have a lot of promise although it's in the very early stages.

202

Our particular study involves stem cells that are isolated from the bone marrow, grown in the laboratory and then reinjected into the MS patient. The stem cells that we give back in large numbers may have the ability to modulate the immune system or migrate into areas of damage and promote repair and that's the premise of our study. There is an abundance of studies in other tissue injuries where they have the ability to do those things. They're being looked at in several immune conditions including MS.

Dr. Cohen admitted that it is understandable that anyone with MS could become somewhat less optimistic when he or she hears a diagnosis of MS. "It is an upsetting diagnosis to receive, but our ability to diagnose the disease, to manage symptoms, to predict how someone's going to do, to treat the disease and to prevent disability is improving year by year. So things look very hopeful."

Following the Research

The message here, obviously, is that not only your treating physician has to be vigilant in watching for changes in clinical protocols and trials, but also you should be seeking out information. Being aware and able to knowledgeably discuss treatment alternatives not only can help you to better understand the disease and the current state of the science around it, but it also enables you to maintain your sense of hope about change. Find the Internet sites that seem most useful to you and visit them regularly. As I mentioned before, be sure you get on whatever really simple syndication (RSS) feeds there are, put yourself on electronic mailing lists or forums, and become actively involved in MS groups. These groups are the ones that researchers often contact when there are new treatments and where presentations will be made on new breakthroughs.

Keep yourself involved in any computer social networking sites that are devoted to MS because this can also be an instant notification of information that can help you. These social networking sites, in fact, have made it possible for researchers and patients to quickly communicate, almost instantaneously, with each other and this has added to quick dissemination of news.

Prior to these Internet services, the only thing you had was the evening news or monthly bulletins or magazines. Now you're right on top of things. Read everything you can and this is one excellent way of combating any fear you may have. Communicate freely with whomever you think might have something you need to know or to whom you wish to contribute information. The larger the network, the better for everyone involved.

Joining the Fight

If you can, don't sit on the sidelines because one of the best ways to combat the depression, anxiety, and mood shifts you'll be feeling as well as the dispirited feeling you can undergo is to remain active. The less active you are, the worse you'll feel. Go out and meet people in the organizations, get involved in fund-raising events, socialize as much as you feel you can, and remain involved in your own life and that of others. Friends and social connections we know are extremely helpful in terms of your mental and physical health. You've heard the interviewees in this book all speak glowingly about their social connections.

All of these things help you to maintain your emotional and psychological balance, so do it. No one said you had to run a long race or stand/sit for hours manning an information table. There are lots of things to do, and someone will help you find a pursuit that is within your ability level. In the process, you'll meet people who will inspire and encourage you, maybe as you've never been inspired before. You'll never know if you don't go out and meet them. You'll also never know how much you can truly do if you don't try to explore something you've never tried before. Skills that you have and of which you really weren't aware may suddenly become evident to your surprise and delight.

Helping others is also one of the ways that will build up your sense of competence again. The reward that you'll receive will be immeasurable and it can be incredibly energizing. Leave "the ugly twins" behind you and learn to laugh again.

Don't just put this book down now that you've finished it; this is the beginning, not the end. Head straight to your computer or your phone and take some action right now. Reach out for today and all your tomorrows, and make each one of them more rewarding, more meaningful, and full of more pleasant accomplishments than you've ever dreamed of. When you do this, you do what? You turn something upsetting (bad) into something good.

Be well.

Further Reading

Cohen JA, Rudick RA, eds. *Multiple Sclerosis Therapeutics*. 3rd ed. London, England: Informa Healthcare; 2007.

Appendix A

The Social Readjustment Rating Scale

LIFE EVENT	VALUE
Death of a spouse	100
Divorce	73
Marital separation	65
Imprisonment	63
Death of a close family member	63
Personal injury or illness	53
Marriage	50
Dismissal from work	47
Marital reconciliation	45
Retirement	45
Change in health of family member	44
Pregnancy	40
Sexual difficulties	39
Gain a new family member	39
Business readjustment	39
Change in financial state	38
Change in frequency of arguments	35
Major mortgage	32
Foreclosure of mortgage or loan	30
Change in responsibilities at work	29
Child leaving home	29
Trouble with in-laws	29
Outstanding personal achievement	28
Spouse starts or stops work	26
Begin or end school	26
Change in living conditions	25
Revision of personal habits	24

Trouble with boss	23
Change in working hours or conditions	20
Change in residence	20
Change in schools	20
Change in recreation	19
Change in church activities	19
Change in social activities	18
Minor mortgage or loan	17
Change in sleeping habits	16
Change in number of family reunions	15
Change in eating habits	15
Vacation	13
Christmas	12
Minor violation of law	11

Used with permission of Dr. Richard Rahe.

Appendix B

Quality of Life Scale

Read each item and **select the number that best describes how satisfied you *are at this time.*** Answer each item even if you do not currently participate in an activity or have a relationship.

7 = delighted
6 = pleased
5 = mostly satisfied
4 = mixed
3 = mostly dissatisfied
2 = unhappy
1 = terrible

1. Material comforts like home, food, convenience, financial security _____

2. Health—being physically fit and vigorous _____

3. Relationships with parents, siblings, other relatives who are communicating, visiting, and helping _____

4. Having and rearing children _____

5. Close relationships with spouse or significant other _____

6. Close friends _____

7. Helping and encouraging others, volunteering, giving advice _____

8. Participating in organizations and public affairs _____

9. Learning—attending school, improving understanding, getting additional knowledge _____

10. Understanding yourself—knowing your assets and limitations—knowing what life is _____

11. Work—job or in home _____

12. Expressing yourself creatively _____

13. Socializing—meeting other people, doing things, parties, and so forth _____

14. Reading, listening to music, or observing entertainment _____

15. Participating in active recreation _____

16. Independence, doing for yourself _____

SCORE: _____

From Burckhardt CS, Anderson KL. The quality of life scale: reliability and utilization. *Health Qual Life Outcomes* [serial online]. October 2003;1(60). Available at: http://www.uib.no/isf/people/doc/qol/qol.pdf. Accessed March 9, 2010.

Appendix C

Daily Exercise Chart

Week day	Exercise	Place	Amount of time	Notes/tips

Week day	Exercise	Place	Amount of time	Notes/tips

Resources

Accelerated Cure Project for Multiple Sclerosis. http://www.acceleratedcure.org/

American Autoimmune Related Diseases Association. http://www.aarda.org

Doctor's Guide, Personal Edition. Multiple Sclerosis. Available at: http://www.docguide.com/news/content.nsf/PatientResAllCateg/Multiple%20Sclerosis?OpenDocument. Accessed December 2009.

Epocrates Online [drug and disease reference]. http://online.epocrates.com/

Gingold, JN. *Facing the Cognitive Challenges of Multiple Sclerosis*. New York, NY: Demos Medical Publishing, LLC; 2006.

Gingold, JN. *Mental Sharpening Stones: Manage the Cognitive Challenges of Multiple Sclerosis*. New York, NY: Demos Medical Publishing, LLC; 2009.

Health Guide. Multiple sclerosis. *New York Times*. December 30, 2009. Available at: http://health.nytimes.com/health/guides/disease/multiple-sclerosis/overview.html. Accessed December 2009.

Internet Disability Resources. Multiple sclerosis. Available at: http://www.netreach.net/~abrejcha/ms.htm. Accessed December 2009.

Lifehacker [computer freeware and free computer tips]. http://lifehacker.com/search/freeware/

MindTools. The link and story methods: remembering a simple list. Available at: http://www.mindtools.com/pages/article/newTIM_01.htm. Accessed December 26, 2009.

MS Trust StayingSmart. www.stayingsmart.org.uk

Multiple Sclerosis Association of America. http://www.msassociation.org

Multiple Sclerosis Foundation. http://www.msfocus.org

MyBrain Games. The Medical Technology Collaborative. www.Mymsmyway.com

Myles R. Loosening the knots of cognitive problems. Inside MS. http://www.nationalmssociety.org/download.aspx?id=116.

National Ataxia Foundation. http://www.ataxia.org

National Institute of Neurological Disorders and Stroke, National Institutes of Health. Multiple sclerosis resources. Available at: http://www.ninds.nih.gov/find_people/voluntary_orgs/vol_org_sub_MS.htm.

National Organization for Rare Disorders. http://www.rarediseases.org

National Multiple Sclerosis Society (March 2008). InsideMS: A special report. MS and the Mind. Available at: http://www.nationalmssociety.org/multimedia-library/.../download.aspx?id=57. Accessed September 15, 2010

National Rehabilitation Information Center. http://www.naric.com

Office of Special Education and Rehabilitative Services. http://www.ed.gov/about/offices/list/osers

Paralyzed Veterans of America. http://www.pva.org

Patients Like Me. http://www.patientslikeme.com/multiple-sclerosis/community

Physical activity guidelines for Americans. Be active your way: a fact sheet for adults. U.S. Department of Health & Human Services Web site. Available at: http://www.health.gov/paguidelines/factSheetAdults.aspx. Accessed December 2009.

Mind Tools, Ltd. Remember! The memory booster workbook, v. 1. Available at: http://www.mindtools.com/downloads/lbr5283hs/RememberWorkbook.pdf. Accessed December 27, 2009.

Montel Williams MS Foundation. http://www.montelms.org/

Turner DL. Notes from a (former) reader. InsideMS, October–December 2004. www.nationalmssociety.org/download.aspx?id=9

U.S. Department of Health & Human Services. Multiple sclerosis. Healthfinder.gov. Available at: http://www.healthfinder.gov/scripts/SearchContext.asp?topic=563. Accessed December 2009.

United States Department of Veterans Affairs. Multiple Sclerosis Center of Excellence. Multiple sclerosis resources. Available at: http://www4.va.gov/MS/multiple-sclerosis-resources.asp.

University of Washington, Rehabilitation Medicine. Multiple Sclerosis Rehabilitation Research and Training Center. http://msrrtc.washington.edu/

WebMD. Multiple sclerosis and resources for caregivers. Available at: http://www.webmd.com/multiple-sclerosis/guide/resources-caregivers. Accessed December 2009.

Well Spouse Association. http://www.wellspouse.org

Index